Public and Community Health Services Requiring Greater Attention

Cognella Series on
Public and Community Health Nursing

Public and Community Health Services Requiring Greater Attention

Anita Finkelman, MSN, RN

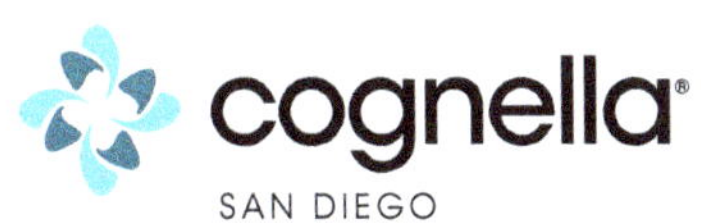

Bassim Hamadeh, CEO and Publisher
Amanda Martin, Publisher
Amy Smith, Senior Project Editor
Rachel Kahn, Production Editor
Emely Villavicencio, Senior Graphic Designer
Kylie Bartolome, Licensing Coordinator
Natalie Piccotti, Director of Marketing
Kassie Graves, Vice President, Editorial
Jamie Giganti, Director of Academic Publishing

Printed in the United States of America.

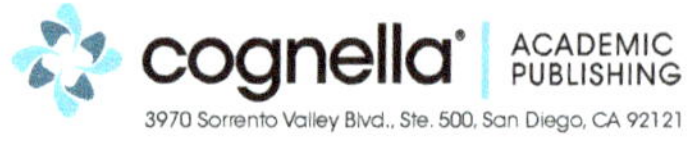

This book is dedicated to all the students who have taught me during my years of professional practice in clinical and academic settings. I also recognize the nurses who have provided care daily during the difficult time of the pandemic, treating all equally in all settings and communities, with special thoughts for those nurses who experienced illness and for those who lost their lives as they worked to improve the health of their communities.

Contents

ACTIVE LEARNING

This book has interactive activities available to complement your reading.

Your instructor may have customized the selection of activities available for your unique course. Please check with your professor to verify whether your class will access this content through the Cognella Active Learning portal (http://active.cognella.com) or through your home learning management system.

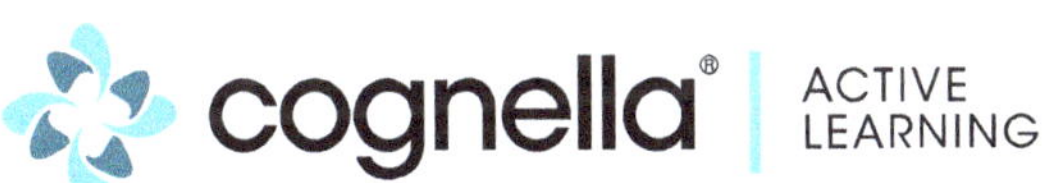

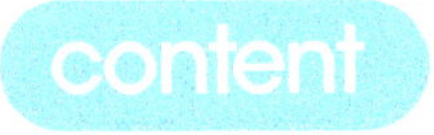

Preface

Due to the COVID-19 pandemic there is a greater recognition of the need for effective public and community health services and for healthcare providers to be more aware of this area of health. This book focuses on improving public and community health and emphasizes this area of healthcare, as well as acute care, as integral to healthcare delivery. Public health services are not only needed during public health emergencies, but at all times and in all communities.

Designed to support current standards and goals for the nursing profession, *Public and Community Health Services Requiring Greater Attention* provides a view of public and community health services that requires an interprofessional team of healthcare providers and others who provide social and community services, while considering the social determinants of health, equity, diversity and disparities, population health, and vulnerable populations.

Public and Community Health Services Requiring Greater Attention is part of the Cognella Series on Public and Community Health Nursing, a collection of concise, informative guides that explores critical topical areas, their nursing applications, and their relationship to nursing practice.

Acknowledgments

I thank my family for their support of my writing and professional endeavors over many years: Fred, Shoshannah, and Deborah, and especially my grandson, Matanel Yizhar, who teaches me daily that learning is constant as well as caring. Thank you to Amanda Martin, a long-time publishing colleague who reached out to me to develop this project. The Cognella team cannot be praised enough for their professionalism and creativity: thanks to Amy Smith for her editing guidance and for keeping me on track; Rachel Kahn for her production leadership; Dani Gradisher, Haley Brown, and all of the others who helped with the development of methods supporting creative student engagement in learning and effective faculty resources; Jeanine Rees for guiding production; Natalie Piccotti, who leads the marketing team; and so many others who have helped with this project behind the scenes.

Public and Community Health Services Requiring Greater Attention

Learning Outcomes

1. Apply the public health framework to support public and community health services.
2. Integrate population health into nursing practice in public/community health services.
3. Compare the types of public and community health services.
4. Examine public and community health services and their relationship to social determinants of health, health equity, diversity and disparities, and vulnerable populations.
5. Compare local, state, and federal government involvement in providing public and community health services.
6. Formulate a summary statement highlighting key points about public and community health services that involve nurses and other healthcare providers in ensuring effective public and community health and health equity.

Key Terms

Case management
Disease prevention
Health disparities
Health equity
Health literacy
Health promotion
Population health management
Social determinants of health (SDOH)
Vulnerable populations

Introduction

The content in this guide focuses on public and community health services, emphasizing population health that considers the social determinants of health (SDOH), health equity, diversity and disparities, and vulnerable populations. The health services examined are those in which nurses participate in a variety of roles and collaborate and coordinate with interprofessional teams. Public and community health is guided by government at all levels, local, state, and national, and engages a range of healthcare providers.

Public Health Framework Supporting Public and Community Health Services

What is public health, and what services does it include? Public health focuses on promoting the health of individuals and communities by emphasizing wellness and healthy behaviors. Its goal is to prevent people from getting sick when possible (APHA, 2021a). Given the range of health and social services needed, effective outcomes require the involvement of multiple providers. Public health should save money in the healthcare system and for individuals and communities. It includes conducting research relevant to these needs and services, providing effective evidence-based interventions, developing plans (such as for public heath emergencies), educating and communicating with the public about health, and maintaining public health organizations to ensure goals are met. At the federal level, the U.S. Department of Health and Human Services (HHS) guides the nation's public and community health. The Centers for Disease Control and Prevention (CDC) outlines 10 essential public health services that "provide a framework for public health to protect and promote the health of *all people in all communities*. To achieve equity, the Essential Public Health Services actively promote policies, systems, and overall community conditions that enable optimal health for all and seek to remove systemic and structural barriers that have resulted in health inequities. Such barriers include poverty, racism, gender discrimination, ableism, and other forms of oppression. Everyone should have a fair and just opportunity to achieve optimal health and well-being" (CDC, 2020). This is the framework that is emphasized in this discussion of public and community health services.

Public health is the area of health care that recognizes the importance of the prevention and control of disease and disability, with particular concern for groups (e.g., populations and communities). Healthy behaviors and wellness are important for public health, and various terms are used to identify those who need public and community health assistance. Examples of these terms include the following:

- individuals (e.g., patients, clients, and consumers)
- families

- aggregates or populations
- communities

There are 3 core public health functions that are related to the 10 essential public health services and are noted below (CDC, 2020):

1. *Assessment:* Relates to essential services 1–2
2. *Policy development:* Relates to essential services 3–5
3. *Assurance:* Relates to essential services 6–10

Nurses who work in public and community health are involved in the three core functions and the following ten essential public health services:

1. "Assess and monitor population health status, factors that influence health, and community needs and assets.
2. Investigate, diagnose, and address health problems and hazards affecting the population.
3. Communicate effectively to inform and educate people about health, factors that influence it, and how to improve it.
4. Strengthen, support, and mobilize communities and partnerships to improve health.
5. Create, champion, and implement policies, plans, and laws that impact health.
6. Utilize legal and regulatory actions designed to improve and protect the public's health.
7. Assure an effective system that enables equitable access to the individual services and care needed to be healthy.
8. Build and support a diverse and skilled public health workforce.
9. Improve and innovate public health functions through ongoing evaluation, research, and continuous quality improvement.
10. Build and maintain a strong organizational infrastructure for public health." (CDC, 2020)

Figure 1 describes the interrelationship between the core functions and essential services.

It is important to distinguish between acute care services and public health services, though they are both parts of the healthcare system. To maintain an effective healthcare system requires collaboration between and coordination of acute and public healthcare services. Acute care focuses on health care for people who are sick or injured and require diagnosis and treatment. Public health services, as noted earlier, focus on protecting and

Centers for Disease Control and Prevention (CDC), "10 Essential Public Health Services," https://www.cdc.gov/publichealthgateway/publichealthservices/essentialhealthservices.html, 2020.

promoting the health of all populations. **Figure 2** describes collaboration in the healthcare system and the community.

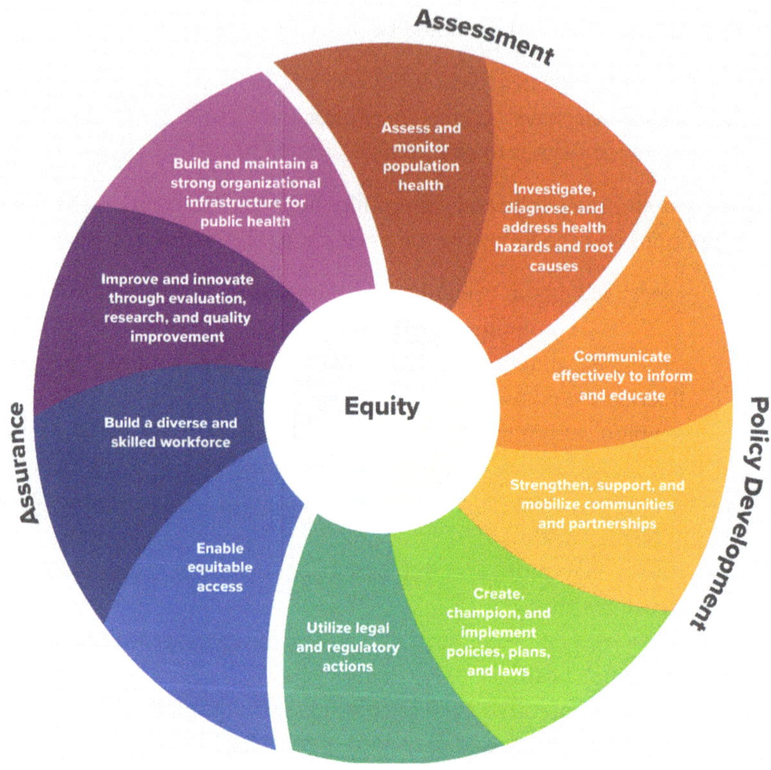

Figure 1. Public Health Core Functions and Essential Services

Population Health in Public and Community Health: Relationship to Services

Public and community health services focus on population health, which is the health of entire populations rather than individual health. This section examines the population health management (PHM) framework and provides examples of public health needs and services.

WHO
Collaborate with Others to Maximize Efforts
PEOPLE
NONPROFITS
COMMUNITY DEVELOPERS
HEALTH INSURANCE
BUSINESSES
COLLECTIVE VISION
PUBLIC HEALTH
EDUCATION
HEALTH CARE PROVIDERS
GOVERNMENT
FAITH-BASED ORGANIZATIONS
PHILANTHROPISTS & INVESTORS

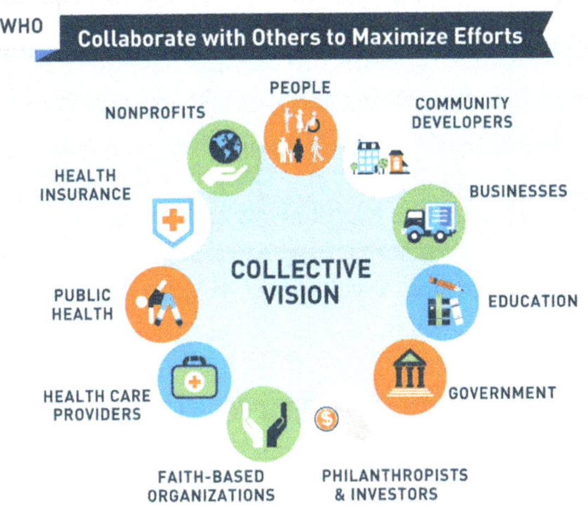

Figure 2. Collaborate With Others to Maximize Efforts

Population Health Management: Frameworks and Key Concepts

Public and community health are key to effective population health; however, as noted above, both parts of the healthcare system need to work together. PHM supports the "triple aim": health of communities, better care, and more affordable care. **Population health management** focuses on populations or groups "within a specific geopolitical area and recognizes that the health of a population is more than just the clinical aspects of care and includes social, economic, environmental, and individual behavioral and genetic traits" (NACHC, 2016). PHM activities relate to improving health across the life span for all populations and include general health; disease management; dental, eye, and hearing treatment; medications and pharmaceutical needs; nutrition; physical therapy and other types of therapies; mental health and substance use treatment; and other areas of healthcare concerns. These activities are recognized as important by the federal government and are supported through government initiatives such as the CDC Division of Population Health (DPH), which offers public health programs, services, resources, and applied research activities (CDC, 2021a). To meet PHM goals requires an effective public and community health process, strategies and planning, and evaluation, which must include consideration of health equity from a population perspective. This requires the following activities (NCQA, 2019):

- *Population analysis:* Data collection and analysis to better understand risks, needs, and outcomes for specific populations
- *Clinical integration:* Healthcare services based on population needs such as immunizations, health screenings, and care focused on specific needs such as hypertension or diabetes
- *Care management/coordination:* Team-based, patient-centered care focused on population health needs and management
- *Patient engagement:* Active support of population (e.g., individuals, families, and groups) involvement in healthcare decision-making, planning, implementation, and evaluation
- *Telehealth integration:* Use of technology to provide, monitor, and document health; includes population involvement either as individuals or groups
- *Claims management:* Process of identifying and ensuring payment for services

Population health management also requires data collection and measurement to determine outcomes. Measurement is focused on the Triple Aim (improve individual health, improve population health, reduce costs) and STEEEP®, the six aims of improvement (safe, timely, effective, efficient, equitable, and patient-centered). PHM requires the involvement of many different healthcare providers and settings, as discussed in the following sections.

Examples of Public Health Needs and Strategies

Public health must be concerned with community health improvement (CHI). This requires an understanding of the who, what, where, and how of improving community health; use of collaborative approaches to establish and maintain effective collaborations; and implementation of interventions for the greatest impact on health and well-being for all in the community (CDC, 2015; HHS Press Office, 2022f). In addition to collaboration, coordination and communication are critical elements of PHM during assessment, planning, implementation, and evaluation of services.

The CDC provides resources for community health improvement as described in **Figures 2–5**. This approach focuses on the following:

1. *What* affects health? (Figure 3)
2. *Where* are the vulnerable populations at greatest risk? (Figure 4)
3. *Who* should you collaborate with to create a plan and reach effective outcomes? (Figure 2)
4. *How* will you implement evidence-based interventions to meet all these areas of concern? (Figure 5)

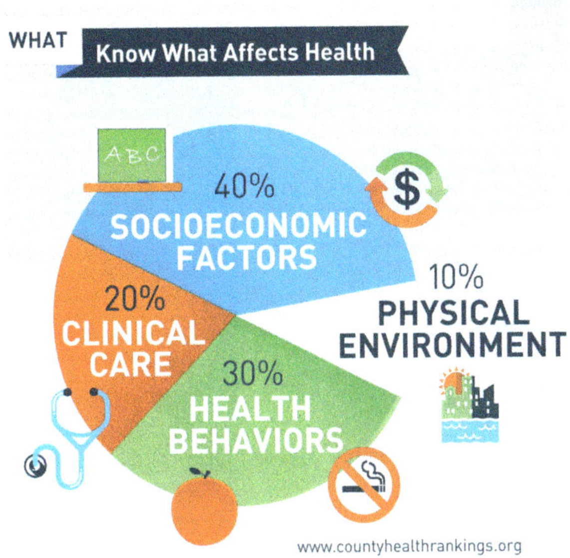

Figure 3. What Affects Health?

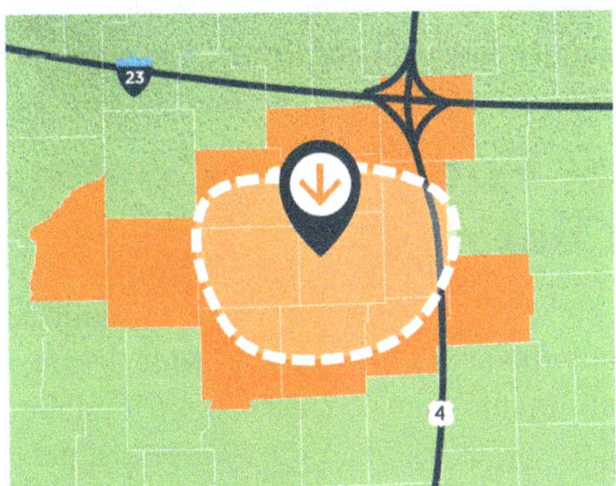

Figure 4. Focus on Areas of Greatest Need

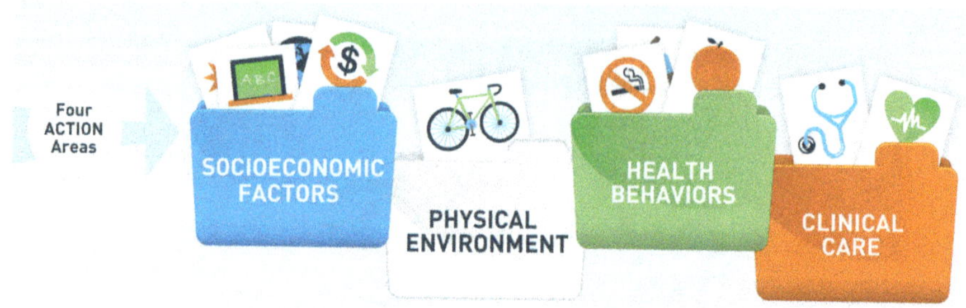

Figure 5. Action Areas

Examples of community needs that require assessment and interventions are:

- water and food safety
- general environmental safety
- infrastructure support, such as electricity and transportation
- communicable diseases—surveillance, public education, immunizations, prevention, and treatment interventions
- leisure and exercise activities and settings such as parks
- available levels of health care and effective post-hospital discharge support in the community

To ensure needs are met requires an understanding of the community through assessment, collection of data, analysis, and planning interventions, which are maintained and improved as needed. Relevant stakeholders and community residents should be included in assessment and planning to improve community outcomes and PHM.

Types of Public and Community Health Services

Effective public and community health services require healthcare providers and other staff who are prepared to provide services. A collaborative of 24 national organizations concerned with public health education developed competencies based on the 10 essential public health services, recommending the application of the competencies for all public health professionals. The goal for this collaboration is to improve public health by ensuring competent staff and effective healthcare organization performance.

Identification of these competencies also recognizes the need for effective coordination and monitoring of outcomes among the key stakeholders in academic institutions, public health practice, healthcare organizations, and communities. Healthcare education must include not only preparation education for healthcare providers but also ongoing staff education at the work site, which should have an interprofessional focus. There is an ongoing need to develop effective strategies for positive public health outcomes; for example, the COVID-19 pandemic required healthcare staff education to ensure understanding and effective application of public health regulations and interventions to keep staff, patients, and community residents safe. The following describes the skills for each of the eight core competencies, or specific activity areas (Council on Linkages between Academia and Public Health Practice, 2021):

1. *Data Analytics and Assessment*

   Focuses on factors that affect the health of the community, data collection, analysis of data, use of public health informatics to inform community members and assess community health status

2. *Policy Development and Program Planning*

   Development, implementation, and evaluation of policies, programs, and services

3. *Communication*

   Internal and external communication, including responding to information (as well as misinformation and disinformation) and facilitating individual, group, and organizational communication

4. *Health Equity*

   Ethics, diversity, equity, inclusion, and justice; self-awareness of biases; working effectively in diverse situations and with diverse people; reducing systematic and structural barriers while advocating for health equity

5. *Community Partnership*

   Establishing community relationships and collaboration to improve community health and resilience; sharing power

6. *Public Health Science*

   Application of essential public health services, evidence-based practice, and support research

7. *Management and Finance*

   Application of basic management and finance skills to public health, including planning, quality, human resources, staff development, finance, policies, integration of diversity, teams and teamwork, collaboration, and performance management; using the healthy community model

8. *Leadership and Systems*

   Identification of facilitators of and barriers to essential public health services; leadership to support creativity, and innovation; responding to current trends, directing effective change, collaborating with community stakeholders, and advocating for public health

In addition to these competencies, all healthcare providers must also follow their own relevant professional standards and competencies. For example, the nursing profession responded to the development of the above core competencies by aligning public health nursing competencies with them. The nursing competencies focus on public health nursing practice, from entry level to all levels of nursing management, and integrate the public health professional core competencies. There are also eight domains in the public health nursing competencies. Given that it is important for public health services to consider health equity and disparities, domains that are particularly related to these issues are identified as follows, although many of the other domains are indirectly related to these issues (Quad Council Coalition, 2018):

- "Cultural competency skills focus on understanding and responding to diverse needs, assessing organizational cultural diversity and competence, assessing effects of policies and programs on different populations, and taking action to support a diverse public health workforce" (p. 21).
- "Community dimensions of practice skills focus on evaluating and developing linkages and relationships within the community, maintaining and advancing partnerships and community involvement, negotiating for the use of community assets, defending public health policies and programs, and evaluating and improving the effectiveness of community engagement" (p. 23).

Healthcare providers are individuals and organizations that provide health services. Examples of individuals are professionals and staff such as physicians, registered nurses, pharmacists, dentists, social workers, nutritionists, psychologists, government health inspectors (food, business safety), health educators, community planners, epidemiologists, public policymakers and planners, school staff, community first responders, occupational health and safety professionals, sanitarians, health educators, public health department management, health technology and informatics staff, and public health researchers (APHA, 2021b).

A staff member who works in public and community health, and rarely in acute health, is the community health worker (CHW), which is a broad term used to describe someone who provides community or public health services. A CHW may or may not be a healthcare professional. They assist in providing community outreach and support, advocacy, health education, and coordination of services in the community. CHWs may be associated with any public health service setting. If they are not a healthcare professional, CHWs receive public health training for this role (APHA, 2021b). The U.S. Department of Health and Human Services (HHS) provides funding for this training. For example, HRSA is increasing its training to develop 13,000 community health workers. This increase in staff should increase access to care, improve public health emergency response, and provide services to meet the public health needs of underserved communities (HHS Press Office, 2022a).

The healthcare system, encompassing acute care and public and community health, includes many different types of healthcare organizations such as acute care hospitals, clinics, community-based service agencies, home healthcare agencies, centers providing urgent care and emergency services, pharmacies, and private medical practices. Community health departments and their associated services, such as clinics and often school health, provide critical services to the community and are part of the local government. The following sections provide an overview of public and community health services and clinical sites.

Ambulatory Services

Ambulatory services are provided in outpatient settings. Ownership and management of ambulatory services or clinics vary. They may be owned and managed by a healthcare provider such as a physician or group of physicians and include acute care hospitals, which can be public or private; public health department clinics at both local and state levels; and federal clinics, such as clinics for veterans or Indian Health Services clinics. In the last few years, other types of clinics have been established such as retail, nurse-led/managed clinics, and accountable care organizations, which are discussed in this section. These settings expand healthcare access and may be in urban or rural areas in a variety of locations. They may have a specific service or population focus besides primary care, such as a specialty medical or surgical, mental health, pediatrics, or maternal and child. In general, "the scope of ambulatory care has expanded over the past decade, as the volume and complexity of interventions have expanded. Safe, high-quality ambulatory care requires complex information management and care coordination across multiple settings, especially for patients with chronic illnesses" (AHRQ, 2018).

Ambulatory Care Nursing Conceptual Framework

Review the ambulatory care nursing conceptual framework at the link below, and write a brief description of the framework.

Website: https://www.aaacn.org/practice-resources/what-ambulatory-care-nursing/conceptual-framework

The nursing specialty organization for ambulatory care, the American Academy of Ambulatory Care Nursing (AAACN), describes key characteristics of ambulatory care, which requires critical reasoning and effective clinical judgment. Patient encounters are usually less than 24 hours, may occur at any time of the day depending on the services and access, and may be for one encounter or more. In some cases, when patients require ambulatory care over a long time period, nurses may develop long-term relationships with their patients. The common ambulatory care nursing activities are (AAACN, 2022):

- Provide quality care across the lifespan to individuals, families, caregivers, groups, populations, and communities.
- Interact with patients using a variety of methods, including face-to-face and virtual methods.
- Provide care services (e.g., assessment, identifying patient needs, performing procedures, documenting, patient advocacy, health education and guidance, coordinating care, communicating with the patient and others, evaluating health outcomes).
- Integrate continuity of care throughout the care process, emphasizing implementation of the nursing process, interprofessional collaboration, and coordination of and access to appropriate healthcare services and community resources across the care continuum.
- Provide care in a variety of settings: hospital-based outpatient clinics/ centers, solo or group medical practices, ambulatory surgery and

> diagnostic procedure centers, telehealth services, university and community hospital clinics, military and Veterans Administration settings, nurse-managed clinics, colleges and educational institutions, freestanding community facilities, care coordination organizations, and patients' homes.

The AAACN standards are published in the *Scope and Standards of Practice for Professional Ambulatory Care Nursing* (AAACN, 2017), and standards for the expanding area of telehealth, which is increasing in ambulatory care, appear in *Scope and Standards of Practice for Professional Telehealth Nursing* (AAACN, 2018). The American Nurses Association standards, *Public Health Nursing: Scope & Standards of Practice*, are also applied in ambulatory settings (ANA, 2022).

Primary Care

Primary care is where individuals receive most of their care, including preventive and acute care, chronic disease management, and specialist referrals. This type of care is typically provided by a physician, but now there is greater access to advanced practice nurses and physician assistants for these services. Primary care was not originally connected to public health services except when care was needed for underserved populations. Health care began to show greater concern for social justice and health equity in the 1960s, though it is now recognized that much more needs to be done to improve health access. Changes occurred, including the development of the safety net healthcare system to better ensure health equity and reduce disparities, particularly for populations that have less access to or cannot afford care (Grant, 2012). In some communities, primary care moved from typical medical offices to community-oriented primary care (COPC). According to Grant, this model

> combined public health methods with primary care practice. Instead of only treating individual patients, primary care providers identified community-wide health problems and developed strategies to address them. With COPC, primary care not only would improve individual health but also improve community health and well-being, an essential public health goal. The COPC model proved economically unsustainable but the goal of developing primary care services that contribute to meeting public health goals remained. (2012)

Today, according to Phillips and Bazemore (2010),

> primary care is a foundational element of the U.S. healthcare system and is required to meet our Nation's triple aims of improving quality, containing costs, and improving patient and family experience. Primary care is also critical to ensuring access to health care for all Americans and reducing healthcare disparities. Whether the focus is on the individual, a population, or the healthcare system, good access to primary care is associated with more timely care, better preventive care, avoiding unnecessary care, improved costs, and lower mortality. (p. 806)

Primary care providers may focus on family health, internal medicine, OB-GYN, pediatrics, geriatrics, or other areas, though typically they provide general health services and act as gatekeepers to specialty care and referrals.

The Affordable Care Act of 2010 (ACA), referred to as a comprehensive healthcare reform, has had an impact on primary care and increased focus on preventive care and care provided by a variety of providers. The major goals for this legislation are (HHS, 2022):

- "Make affordable health insurance available to more people. The law provides consumers with subsidies ('premium tax credits') that lower costs for households with incomes between 100% and 400% of the federal poverty level (FPL).
- Expand the Medicaid program to cover all adults with income below 138% of the FPL. Not all states have expanded their Medicaid programs.
- Support innovative medical care delivery methods designed to lower the costs of health care generally."

The law also supports healthcare education, with a focus on primary care, and provides incentives to increase the healthcare workforce in communities that are underserved. The initiative addresses the need for greater primary care access and quality of care, as well as decreased healthcare costs (Brown et al., 2021).

It has been just over 10 years since this law was passed. What have been the outcomes? The ACA has reduced the number of uninsured, particularly for economically marginalized groups and people of color, but there have been changes and legal threats to this law. Additionally, "the law's effects on the cost and quality of healthcare services are difficult to discern given the complexity of our health system" (Blumenthal et al., 2020). There is a need for continuing evaluation of the outcomes, and if changes need to be made, they will need to be addressed through updates to the law.

Primary Care Medical Home

Another change that occurred in public and community health was the establishment of the primary care medical home model (PCMH). The PCMH core functions are (AHRQ, 2022a):

1. *Comprehensive care:* Physical and mental healthcare needs for prevention and wellness, acute care, and chronic care; provided by interprofessional team (physicians, advanced practice nurses, physician assistants, nurses, pharmacists, nutritionists, social workers, educators, and care coordinators)
2. *Patient-centered care* (or *person-centered care*): Relationship-based care focused on the whole person, developing partnerships with patients and their families, and understanding and respecting each patient's unique needs, culture, values, and preferences; using effective communication; supporting self-management and patient health education
3. *Accessible services:* Providing services that increase access, such as hours of service, around-the-clock advice (telephone and electronic), and easy access to parking and transportation
4. *Quality and safety:* Evaluation and application of methods to improve care such as using evidence-based practice (EBP), collecting data and monitoring health outcomes, collecting patient feedback and applying it to improve care (when possible), and applying standards of care and management

Nurse Managed Health Centers

Nurse managed health centers (NMHC) focus on health care for the more than 46 million people who do not have health insurance and communities that are underserved in both urban and rural areas. The services they provide are primary care, health promotion, and disease prevention. There are over 200 NMHCs serving 2.5 million patients (AAN, 2021). Many of the NMHCs are associated with schools of nursing in their communities. They are also used as clinical education sites with participating faculty for nursing students and nurse practitioners. These centers focus on health equity and reducing health disparities and are designated as safety-net providers by the federal government (Bagwell et al., 2017). Outcomes from these centers have been very positive, and include lower hospitalization rates, greater use of generic medications that reduces costs, and positive health outcomes.

Accountable Care Organizations

The Centers for Medicare and Medicaid Services (CMS) defines accountable care organizations (ACOs) as

> groups of doctors, hospitals, and other healthcare providers, who come together voluntarily to give coordinated high-quality care to the Medicare patients they serve. Coordinated care helps ensure that patients, especially the chronically ill, get the right care at the right time, with the goal of avoiding unnecessary duplication of services and preventing medical errors. When an ACO succeeds in both delivering high-quality care and spending healthcare dollars more wisely, it will share in the savings it achieves for the Medicare program. (2022a)

ACOs use community partnerships to ensure access to effective care and emphasize patient or Medicare beneficiary needs and preferences. They also use data to improve performance and quality of care. ACOs were first established in 2012, emphasizing coordination, patient engagement, and provider engagement as key values (CMS, 2021). ACOs identify patients who are at higher risk early so that they receive the care they need and use interprofessional teams. These clinics also use case managers, who are usually registered nurses, to coordinate care to ensure health and wellness and consider critical factors related to chronic disease management, social determinants of health, and health promotion and behavior modification (Day et al., 2022).

Retail Clinics

Retail clinics are now found in many communities. They are primary care clinics located in settings that offer easy access in sites that are often used by consumers such as shopping malls, grocery stores, and pharmacies (AAFP, 2022). Their services may include preventive care, immunizations, and physical exams (such as for children's sport activities, and common medical testing), and care for less complex illnesses. Hours are typically broad, including days, evenings, and weekends, and appointments are often not required. These clinics have varied ownership; for example, hospitals or the site where the clinic is located such as a pharmacy may own and manage the clinic. The most common staff are advanced practice nurses under physician supervision and consultation. Hospitals that own these clinics expect referrals from the clinics.

Urgent Care Centers

Urgent care centers are found in many communities. This type of center is not the same as a retail clinic, though both focus on easy access (Heath,

2017). Urgent care centers provide care for medical problems that are urgent but not life-threatening. These centers are not the same as hospital emergency departments, which can handle a broad range of needs and levels of care. Often patients can receive care faster in urgent care centers than they would in an emergency department where less acute emergencies may not be addressed as quickly. Urgent care centers also reduce emergency department workload as they receive patients who do not require emergency level services. Urgent care centers are convenient and cost effective. Examples of some health problems that can be addressed in urgent care settings are sprains, urinary tract infections, fever, flu, mild or moderate asthma, minor accidents and falls, and lacerations. Patients may not be clear about whether they should go to a community urgent care center or emergency department. After an assessment, staff may need to assist in this decision. Communities should prepare educational materials for the public to better understand their choices when they need urgent or emergency care to reduce overuse of emergency services and direct community members to other types of public and community health settings such as an urgent care when they face urgent but less acute medical problems.

Community Health Centers

The community health center (CHC) model is one of the largest U.S. primary and preventive care services. CHCs are private, nonprofit, or public entities, including tribal and faith-based organizations, that operate under the direction of a patient-majority governing board. They are found in many states. They provide

> comprehensive, culturally competent, high-quality primary healthcare services to the nation's most vulnerable individuals and families, including people experiencing homelessness, agricultural workers, residents of public housing, and veterans. Health centers integrate access to pharmacy, mental health, substance use disorders, and oral health services in areas where there are economic, geographic, or cultural barriers that limit access to affordable health care. By emphasizing coordinated care management of patients with multiple healthcare needs and the use of key quality improvement practices, including health information technology, health centers reduce health disparities. (HRSA, 2021b)

Human Resources and Services Administration (HRSA), "What is a Health Center?" https://bphc.hrsa.gov/about-health-centers/what-health-center, 2021.

Ability to pay should not limit access, and some care may be provided on a sliding scale, often to people from diverse backgrounds and to under-resourced communities. Some community health centers focus on specific populations such as individuals and families experiencing homelessness, migratory and seasonal agricultural workers, and residents of public housing. These centers offer the following to members of the community (HRSA, 2021b):

- comprehensive, culturally competent, high-quality primary health care, as well as supportive services such as health education, translation, and transportation
- services regardless of patients' ability to pay and based on a sliding fee scale
- systems of patient-centered (person-centered) and integrated care that responds to the unique needs of diverse populations

In August 2022, President Biden approved funding for the American Rescue Plan for the Health Resources and Services Administration (HRSA), which is part of the HHS. This funding awarded an estimated $90 million to nearly 1,400 community health centers to support health equity through better data collection (HHS Press Office, 2022a; HHS Press Office, 2022b). More than 30 million people benefit from CHC services, and these services greatly impact public and community health outcomes. This funding was announced in conjunction with the government's proclamation about National Health Center Week. "HRSA's initiative is designed to enable health centers to have better data on both patient health status and social determinants of health. With better information, programs can tailor their efforts to improve health outcomes and advance health equity by more precisely targeting the needs of specific communities or patients, particularly as part of the public health emergency response" (HHS Press Office, 2022e).

CHCs provide medical, dental, and behavioral health services. They often serve populations and communities with limited healthcare access but are also important during public health emergencies such as COVID-19. CHCs provide health care to 1 in 5 people living in rural communities, and 1 in 11 people nationwide. More than 90% of HRSA-funded CHC patients are individuals or families living at or below 200% of the Federal Poverty Guidelines, and nearly 63% are from racial or ethnic minorities. The HHS is developing more effective data-driven approaches to assist programs such as CHCs to be more effective. These programs are "designed to collect more and better data on social determinants of health, while also streamlining and improving data quality reporting for health centers. This effort will enable health centers to tailor their efforts to improve health outcomes and advance health equity, more precisely targeting the needs of specific communities or patients. Health centers are vital to increasing equitable access to primary health care" (HHS Press Office, 2022b). CHCs are part of expanded initiatives focused on health equity and the need to assess outcomes to improve public and community health services.

Community Health Centers

Find your state and review its activity related to CHC funding.

Website: https://bphc.hrsa.gov/funding/funding-opportunities/arp-uds-supplemental-funding/awards

Review general information about the HRSA Health Center Program.

Website: https://bphc.hrsa.gov/about-health-centers

Mobile Health Clinics

Mobile health clinics are available in some communities to bring primary care and prevention services, such as immunizations, mammograms, and well child services, to those who need these services. Nursing students, other healthcare profession students, and their faculty may be involved in providing services in these clinics. A recent study of these clinics indicates they serve many vulnerable populations with:

> a median number of 3,491 visits annually. More than half of their clients are women (55%) and racial/ethnic minorities (59%). Of the 146 clinics that reported insurance data, 41% of clients were uninsured while 44% had some form of public insurance. The most common service models were primary care (41%) and prevention (47%). With regards to organizational affiliations, they vary from independent (33%) to university affiliated (24%), while some (29%) are part of a hospital or health care system. (Malone et al., 2020)

Health Promotion and Prevention Services

Public health addresses **health promotion** and prevention. As communities assess their health needs, they must analyze how they promote and support healthy lifestyles. This assessment needs to consider nutrition (e.g., access to healthy foods, types of restaurant choices people have, school meals including free breakfasts for children with limited access to food, and health education on nutrition and safe dieting). Exercise is also part of a community response to health promotion (e.g., access to safe and clean parks, playgrounds, and public exercise areas such as bike paths, jogging areas, swimming pools, and gyms). Health promotion strategies need to consider health equity and the community's diversity. Communities may also provide access to stress management activities; for example, community centers and schools may offer classes in stress management. However, plans for these activities need to consider cost, location, and reasonable hours to ensure access and health equity. Primary care providers in all types of settings should offer stress assessments and make recommendations when needed to improve stress management for their patients. Communities should consider these needs when developing health education materials and activities for their community and identify different population needs based on housing, economics, language, culture, religion, age, and residential locations that may impact stress.

Community Pharmacy Services and Pharmacists

"Pharmacy and public health are a perfect intersection on the healthcare system roadways. Pharmacy and public health have the primary goal of ensuring a population of healthy people" (Mager & Moore, 2020). The typical description of the pharmacist's role is that the pharmacist fills prescriptions; however, there are now expanding views of this role (Chiara, 2022). It is important to recognize that in the United States nearly 9 in 10 people live within 5 miles of a community pharmacy and 4 in 5 have prescription benefits through their health insurance pharmacy benefit manager (PBM), which manages prescription benefits for an insurer and may be used by both private and government insurers such as Medicare Part D drug plans. PBMs focus on reducing drug costs and increasing patient access to medications. They may also represent the insurer in processing prescription claims and negotiating drug costs (Commonwealth Fund, 2019).

Communities are dependent on drugstores or pharmacies and broad service stores such as grocery stores that also have these services for consumers. Typically, they are for-profit businesses, often part of a chain. Hospitals may also have pharmacies open to the public, but this is less common. Up until recently, prescriptions were filled at these sites, and most consumers paid for them through some type of health insurance. These pharmacies had collaborative arrangements with insurers. This, however, is changing due to pharmacists realizing that working with insurers for all their payments was complex and not always a positive financial benefit to them or consumers (Kaplan et al., 2022). Some pharmacists are starting cash pharmacies where they do not accept insurance for payment. It is common to think that insurance helps consumers pay for services, but in some cases with medications the consumer is paying more for medications if using insurance coverage and some insurance plans may have prescription limits. Why is this? Using insurance to pay for name-brand medications without generic options is still the best choice. The "cash" or "self-pay" pharmacies offer more generic drug options that are cheaper as they buy them wholesale with a small increase in cost to the consumer. Even when the cost of insurance is considered, generic drugs may be cheaper. Many drugs needed for chronic conditions and acute problems are safe and effective generic drugs. Even some large companies have begun to offer special options for consumers to obtain generic drugs at lower cost (Kaplan et al., 2022). This is all relatively new, and for most prescriptions consumers continue to pay with insurance coverage. Communities also vary in their options, but public health requires access to all health services, and this includes consideration of costs for medications and medical supplies.

Some of the services pharmacists can provide due to their training are not commonly known, such as blood pressure screening, educating patients with diabetes on the effective use of glucometers, chronic disease management, some medical testing, tobacco cessation, opioid counseling and education, identifying and recommending over-the-counter remedies for common illnesses and decreasing need for doctor visits and costs, emergency preparedness guidance, and health education. Advice about over-the-counter remedies is a service known by many consumers, but the other services are less known and could be used to expand public health services in the community.

Many pharmacies now offer immunizations routinely, usually on walk-in basis. This service has been used for COVID-19 immunizations, and some pharmacies have been involved in COVID-19 testing. In July 2022, the Food and Drug Administration (FDA) issued an emergency authorization allowing pharmacists to prescribe and provide the medication Paxlovid for COVID-19. Use was based on specific criteria, making it more easily available when someone tested positive for COVID-19 and could benefit from taking this drug. They can get the prescription in the same place where testing was done and results received, limiting delays (Center for Drug Evaluation and Research, 2022). Making adaptations like this is very important in public health, eliminating the need for appointments and visits to healthcare facilities but still providing safe, effective care. This type of change may then lead to other more permanent changes.

Another change in pharmacy services that has an impact on public health is obtaining prescriptions online. In these systems consumers can transfer their prescriptions to the online pharmacy site, get prescriptions delivered to their homes, and gain virtual or telephone access pharmacists 24/7 for information. Some pharmacy sites offer maintenance of an electronic personal medication history.

Healthy People 2030, the national health prevention and promotion initiative, recognizes the importance of pharmaceutical services and includes objectives that relate to these services and public health (ODPHP, 2020a):

- Reduce the misuse of drugs and alcohol (substance use disorders).
- Provide immunizations and control of infectious diseases.
- Reduce the inappropriate use of antibiotics.
- Reduce hospitalizations among older adults for diabetes, pneumonia, and urinary tract infections.
- Manage chronic illnesses and diseases including hypertension, diabetes, respiratory, cardiovascular, or renal illnesses and cancer.
- Develop emergency preparedness and response, including for natural disasters.
- Ensure medical product safety, including decreases in emergency room visits for medication overdoses among young children, overdoses from oral anticoagulants, and overdoses from insulin.
- Prevent disease and injury.

See **Appendix A** for more information about Healthy People.

There have been many changes in pharmacy services in last few years, and most likely more will occur. A recent example is the decision by the large national pharmacy chain CVS to purchase a company, Signify Health, that offers physician home visits (Hirsch, 2022). Why would this be done by a pharmacy chain? It is suggested that it might be due to the increasing competition pharmacies are experiencing with consumers using virtual methods to order and receive prescriptions. Signify Health currently has 10,000 physicians that provide in-home visits to 2.5 million patients nationwide, with a focus on Medicare beneficiaries and populations that are underserved. With this partnership, physicians can also direct patients to CVS for prescriptions. Since this is a very new approach, it is not now possible to determine the outcome of this type of arrangement, but it is an example of change that combines multiple services in the community. Even having a physician complete a home visit is not that common. Insurance companies are recognizing more and more that care in the home may reduce the need for inpatient and acute care, and this reduces costs.

School-Based Health

School health is offered in elementary, middle, and high schools, both public and private. School health nurses provide most of the services. Some schools

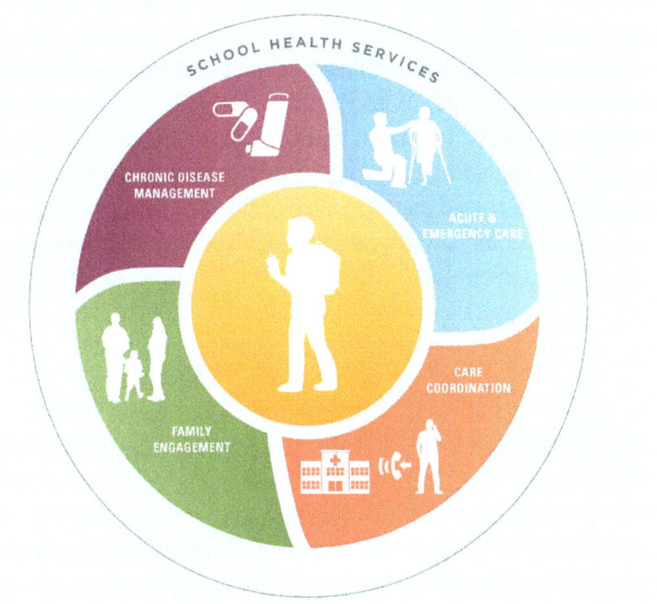

Figure 6. School Health

also use health aides who are supervised by nurses. School health staff may be part of the local public health department. **Figure 6** highlights the key school health functions, and school health services represent a critical component of public health. In some communities, school health nurses, often advanced practice pediatric nurses, offer extensive primary care to children and monitor their health. They serve as resources to the teachers and other staff when they may be concerned about the health of a child or groups of children. They are resources for health information and guidance related to growth and development, as well as emotional concerns and the impact of experiences such as bullying, substance use, nutrition, exercise, and family needs. School nurses also provide assessment, guidance, and referrals for children who have learning disabilities/disorders, working with their teachers and families. It may not be possible for a nurse to be in a school for the entire day, as in some communities nurses may need to cover more than one school due to staffing and budget shortages. Nurses also provide routine interventions and assessment related to eyesight, hearing, and immunizations. During epidemics and pandemics such as COVID-19, nurses need to be aware of public health regulations and assist education staff in implementing regulations to keep students and staff safe. During flu season, school nurses are important in providing health guidance and assessment of children who may be sick and need to be sent home, and this also applies to other infectious diseases that children may experience.

The HHS has provided $25 million to expand school-based health services (HHS Press Office, 2022c). With the impact of COVID-19 on children more support is now needed for them, and this can be included in school-based health services, providing easy and familiar access to assessment and care guidance. With increased mental health problems among children and teens (for example, problems with anxiety and depression), more services are needed. School nurses along with teachers may be able to identify a child in need of help early and then collaborate to get the help the child needs. These services should also partner with other community services, such as social services. "One in nine children in the United States accesses primary health care through a HRSA-funded health center. In 2020, 41 percent of health centers provided services to children and youth at over 3,200 school-based sites" (HHS Press Office, 2022c). School nurses and staff assist in improving health equity and access to health services and work collaboratively with other healthcare providers in the community by developing an effective referral base to meet a variety of needs and working with parents to ensure needs are met.

Occupational Health

Occupational health is a public health service that promotes and maintains physical, mental, and social well-being of workers in all occupations. Its objectives are to promote employee health, improve working environments to ensure work safety, and develop healthy, positive work environments (WHO, 2022a). Occupational health is based on the science and practice of occupational medicine, nursing, ergonomics, psychology, and safety. The types of services that an employee health center might offer are injury care and referral; immunizations; screenings; case management; physical exams; health education; surveillance of injury risk in the workplace; intervention recommendations; and implementation of state and federal health and safety regulations. The World Health Assembly urges countries to develop effective policies and plans focused on occupational health, increase occupational health interventions to reduce work-related injuries and illnesses, and increase collaboration among stakeholders concerned with communicable and noncommunicable diseases, prevention of injuries, health promotion, mental health, environmental health, and health systems development (WHO, 2022a). Occupational health service providers include physicians, nurses, and others depending on the workplace type and size, and employers should be engaged in these efforts.

There are two federal agencies that focus on health and safety in the workplace, the Occupational Safety and Health Administration (OSHA) and the National Institute for Occupational Safety and Health (NIOSH).

Both are federal government agencies that are active nationwide in ensuring workforce health and safety.

The OSHA was established in 1970 as part of the Occupational Safety and Health Act "to ensure safe and healthful working conditions for workers by setting and enforcing standards and by providing training, outreach, education and assistance" (OSHA, 2022). This agency is part of the U.S. Department of Labor. The OSHA focuses on private sector employers and their workers and some from the public sector. Its key functions are the development and implementation of health and safety standards for the workplace, workplace conduct, inspections, and enforcement, as well as the application of penalties when employers fail to meet requirements. To better monitor outcomes, employers with more than 10 employees must document serious work-related injuries and illnesses. Staff responsible for health and safety concerns must follow OSHA record keeping and reporting requirements. The agency provides training resources for employers and employees on a variety of health and safety issues through its website.

The NIOSH is a CDC agency, so it is part of the U.S. Department of Health and Human Services. Its mission and vision are to support "safer, healthier workers; to develop new knowledge in the field of occupational safety and health and to transfer that knowledge into practice," and its strategic plan goals for 2019–2024 include the following (NIOSH, 2022):

1. Reduce occupational cancer, cardiovascular disease, adverse reproductive outcomes, and other chronic diseases.
2. Reduce occupational hearing loss.
3. Reduce occupational immune, infectious, and dermal disease.
4. Reduce occupational musculoskeletal disorders.
5. Reduce occupational respiratory disease.
6. Improve workplace safety to reduce traumatic injuries.
7. Promote safe and healthy work design and well-being.

The NIOSH conducts research to meet its mission and goals. It also provides resources for health and safety in the workplace through its website.

NIOSH and Occupational Health

Review the following link for NIOSH. What are five examples of workplace safety and health topics that the agency focuses on in its resources? Review the five you select.

Website: https://www.cdc.gov/niosh/index.htm

The American Association of Occupational Health Nursing (AAOHN) is a professional organization for nurses who provide health services in the workplace, for example for healthcare organizations (e.g., hospitals), factories, other types of industries, corporations, and so on. "Occupational and environmental health nursing is the specialty practice that provides for and delivers health and safety programs and services to workers, worker populations, and community groups" (AAOHN, 2022). Nurses who work in this area of public health provide healthcare services to promote and restore health, prevent illness and injury, and protect employees from work-related and environmental hazards. Examples of their activities are case management to coordinate care for sick and injured employees; interventions to promote health and prevent illness; counseling for work-related mental health and substance use issues; crisis intervention; assessment of work-related safety and hazard risks; and participation in ensuring workplace regulations, such as those provided by OSHA and, recently, by the CDC on COVID-19, are carried out.

Home Health Care

Services provided in the home have long been available, but as the older population increases, communities have a greater need for these services. Home health care is also needed for people of all ages who have disabilities and complex health problems. These services are provided through home healthcare agencies that may be managed as private or non-profit organizations and hospitals, or may be part of government health services at the local, state, or federal levels.

Some health insurance plans cover home healthcare services. The common criteria for insurance coverage for these services, for example Medicare coverage, are: The patient has a designated healthcare provider for treatment orders and the patient and provider have a face-to-face meeting within 90 days prior to initiation of home care and within 30 days after home care begins; the patient is certified by a recognized provider to be homebound (meaning it is extremely difficult for the patient to leave home) and requires intermittent care (care needed at least once every 60 days and at most once a day for up to three weeks); and skilled nursing care is provided by a professional or under the supervision of a professional (Medicare Interactive, 2022). The following are the common types of home-based care, categorized by the type of services provided and the patient's functional and medical goals of care (McElroy et al., 2022):

1. *Custodial care* constitutes the largest segment of home-based care. It is estimated that more than 21.3% or 53 million Americans were informal caregivers (family or friends or trained paid caregivers)

to either a child or adult in 2020; over half of these provide care to 5.5 million adults, 3.6 million of whom have dementia.

2. *Home health agencies* provide care by employing visiting licensed nurses, home health aides, and physical, occupational, and speech therapists in the patient's place of living.
3. *Home-based primary care* is provided by physicians or advanced practice providers including nurse practitioners, physician assistants, and pharmacists.
4. *Independence at home* (IAH) is a specific type of home-based care service aimed at frail, homebound older adults that was started by CMS to provide comprehensive primary care services to Medicare beneficiaries with multiple chronic conditions.

Medicare Parts A and B includes coverage for home health care services such as (CMS, 2022b)

- part-time or intermittent skilled nursing care
- physical therapy
- occupational therapy
- speech-language pathology services
- medical social services
- part-time or intermittent home health aide care (only if the patient is also getting other skilled services like nursing and/or therapy at the same time)
- administration of injectable osteoporosis drugs for women
- durable medical equipment
- medical supplies for use at home

A home healthcare agency coordinates with the patient's designated provider and agency staff to provide care in the home. This may eliminate the need for hospitalization, reduce inpatient time, or provide long-term care, allowing the patient to stay at home in familiar surroundings. The patient will still need to receive typical services such as personal care, meals, house cleaning, laundry care, and other activities, as these are not covered by insurers such as Medicare or Medicaid. The CMS requires that beneficiaries who receive these services must be homebound but allows the patient to go to medical appointments and leave home for short periods of time and infrequently, such as to participate in religious services, and their care is followed and certified by a physician. The latter CMS requirement has recently changed, and it is an example of a major change that was made due to COVID-19. The CMS changed its approval of providers that could provide home health services without physician certification, expanding it to include nurse practitioners, clinical nurse specialists, and physician assistants (CMS, 2022b). Prior to this change, these providers were involved in providing care, but not in the initiation and maintenance of the care, which required physician approval or certification. Patients participating in adult care day care may receive Medicare home healthcare services, and this is important for many older adults.

The Affordable Care Act of 2010 expanded CMS coverage to Medicaid home healthcare services for Medicaid beneficiaries with two or more chronic illnesses, one chronic illness with risk for a second, or presence of a serious persistent mental health condition. Services that are included are (CMS, 2022a):

- comprehensive care management
- care coordination
- health promotion
- comprehensive transitional care/follow-up
- patient and family support
- referral to community and social support services

Since Medicaid is jointly funded and administered by federal and state governments, there can be differences in payment, services, and approved providers among the states. Medicaid provides health coverage to low-income people and is one of the largest payers for health care in the United States, so it is an important source of support for vulnerable populations.

Caregivers are important members of the healthcare team (Marrelli, 2017a; 2017b). Family members or others identified by the patient or family may be caregivers for someone receiving care in the home. This responsibility can be complex and stressful for the caregivers and may involve providing care and meeting home needs or coordinating with others to do these activities. Communities need to consider the needs of caregivers and collect information about the use of homecare services. Home healthcare agencies are a good source for this information; however, many people are cared for at home without using home healthcare agencies. Community agencies, such as social services, non-profit organizations, healthcare providers, and faith-based organizations, may also have information about the needs in a community. Aspects of daily living are part of these needs, such as food, access to prescriptions and care for other medical needs, housekeeping, financial support and banking/bill payment, psychological support, transportation (to medical appointments or for medical emergencies), communication (access to telephone and other emergency alert systems), safe housing and home repairs, regular check-ins, and plans for care and response during disasters or weather events that may limit electricity and heating. Caregivers themselves need support. Typically, they must provide care and coordinate care over a long time period. While they have these responsibilities, they also have their own personal needs and may even have employment responsibilities. Some caregivers do not live in the same location as the person who needs assistance, for example, family members. They are long-distance caregivers. This makes the process difficult for the person who needs care and support, the healthcare providers, and the caregivers, and requires virtual communication, coordination, and decision-making. With many families living in different cities and states, this is a major public and community health need that often is not addressed.

Long-Distance Caregiving

Review the information provided by the Institute on Aging about long-distance caregiving. How might you use this type of information as a public health nurse?

Website: https://www.nia.nih.gov/health/getting-started-long-distance-caregiving

Palliative Care and Hospice

How are palliative care and hospice care different? “Palliative care eases symptoms of serious illnesses and may accompany treatments to cure the illness, and hospice care provides comfort for patients who are terminally ill and not seeking a cure” (HHS, 2017). Palliative care and hospice care are public health services found in most communities. Both can be provided in the patient’s home or other type of residential setting, at a free-standing site, or in hospital units. Though many people who need these services are older adults, they are provided to people of all ages. In addition, due to the nature of certain illnesses, a caregiver or family member may be very active in the care process and in making care decisions. Whenever possible, the patient should also be engaged in the process. This care may include medical care for symptoms, or palliative care and treatment intended to cure a serious illness. The healthcare service focuses on the person’s quality of life and their family. It is best that palliative care begins soon after diagnosis, providing medical, social, emotional, and practical support in hospitals, the home, clinics, and long-term care facilities. These services may be covered by personal insurance, Medicare, Medicaid, and Veteran’s Affairs. In some situations, it may be determined that the patient may not live longer than six more months, and then care may transition to hospice care.

Hospice care focuses on care for people who are approaching the end of life. “At some point, it may not be possible to cure a serious illness, or a patient may choose not to undergo certain treatments. Hospice is designed for this situation. The patient beginning hospice care understands that his or her illness is not responding to medical attempts to cure it or to slow the disease's progress" (NIA, 2021). The types of services and support provided to the patient, family, or caregivers is like palliative care, though many patients receiving palliative care are not terminally ill. Both palliative care and hospice care emphasize interprofessional teams, collaboration, coordination, communication, and engaging the patient and family in the process. Hospice care may also be covered by the same types of insurance as palliative care and provided in similar settings by similar healthcare providers.

During the COVID-19 pandemic, hospice and palliative care services were under great stress due to heavy workloads and complex problems such as infection control. Public health nurses should recognize that these services may need to be supported more and even expanded during public health emergencies (Kates et al., 2021).

Home health care is an important nursing specialty. The International Home Care Nurses Organization (IHCNO) is one specialty organization for home care nurses. The organization notes that "home care nursing's patients include those with acute or chronic health problems, no matter how young or old. Patients include those receiving hospital-at-home, skilled, private duty and palliative services, and many other types of care provided in the patient's home. We recognize that home care nursing is a specialized area of nursing practice, and we seek to support nurses in home healthcare clinical practice, education, and research" (IHCNO, 2022).

Older Adults and a Variety of Services

"Long-term care involves a variety of services designed to meet a person's health or personal care needs during a short or long period of time. These services help people live as independently and safely as possible when they can no longer perform everyday activities on their own" (NIA, 2017b). These services are provided in a variety of settings and by different healthcare providers. In addition, it is important to include caregivers who may be family members or significant others in the care team. Settings include the home (home health care, hospice care, palliative care), adult day care centers, skilled nursing care centers, nursing homes, and a variety of residential models. Private practice settings and clinics also provide healthcare services in the community. Though the tendency is to think of long-term care as only for older adults, age can vary, and a key factor is the person's health status. Older adults often receive care from several providers, which requires interprofessional teams to coordinate care. It is important that the care is coordinated so that needs are met and to limit adverse events due to communication problems such as lack of information or confusion about what is being done by different providers. Decisions should be made based on current and long-term care needs. One approach that is part of this process emphasizes supporting "aging in place" whenever possible—keeping older adults in their own surroundings provides support and consistency.

Aging in Place

Review the following information on aging in place. How might you use this information in public health?

Website: https://www.nia.nih.gov/health/infographics/aging-place-tips-making-home-safe-and-accessible

More detailed information can be found at https://www.nia.nih.gov/health/what-long-term-care.

There are several terms used to describe long-term care options. The following are some of these terms (NIA, 2017a).

- *Board and care homes:* These are residential care facilities or group homes of 20 or less residents, with private or shared rooms, that provide personal care and meals with staff assistance. Nursing and medical care are not provided.
- *Assisted living*: These are care facilities with 25 to 120 residents, usually in individual apartments or rooms with common shared spaces. There are several levels of care with different fees. Residents need daily care assistance, but the care facility does not provide as much care as a nursing home. Services are broad and may include personal care, medication management, housekeeping and laundry, meals, on-site staff for supervision, and social and recreational activities.
- *Nursing homes:* These may be referred to as skilled nursing facilities, and they provide health services and personal care; meals; housekeeping; social and recreational activities; and physical, occupational and speech therapy. Length of stay can vary.
- *Continuing care* retirement communities (*CCRCs*): These facilities provide all levels of services in one location, including independent living in apartments or houses with the option for residents to transition between the levels of service as need.

Consumer access to affordable medications has long been a problem in public health, and one that impacts all ages and populations. Older adults are particularly at risk of limited access to prescriptions due to financial barriers. As a result, some older adults either do not take the medications they need, or they limit doses to stretch out prescriptions. This can lead to complications and the need for more care. This problem continues to be a major public health concern. A recent report from the National Academy of Medicine, *Making Medicines Affordable: A National Imperative* (NAM, 2018), examines this critical problem from the perspectives of cost, insurance, and other factors. (Examples of other NAM reports are described in **Appendix B.**) In July 2022, President Biden signed the Inflation Reduction Act, which includes several provisions, one of which is the need to reduce prescription drug prices. "This historic legislation will help millions of Medicare enrollees better afford their life-sustaining medications, and millions more Americans will be able to pay Affordable Care Act premiums" (Bunis, 2022). Both changes should improve access to public health. Secretary of HHS Xavier Becerra made the following comments about this new law:

> We all have the right to high-quality, affordable health care. ... With this bill, millions of Americans will see lower health care costs. The Inflation Reduction Act locks in premiums that save 13 million people an average of $800 per year. For anyone who relies on Medicare, the bill will put a $2,000 cap on their out-of-pocket costs for the prescription drugs that they need. In addition, it will do something that we have tried—and failed—to do in Washington for decades—allow Medicare to negotiate a better deal on prescription drugs. No one should have to go without health care or a prescription they need because they can't afford it. (HHS Press Office, 2022d)

Case Management Services

For many years case management has been provided to patients who needed this service, and its use has increased. One possible reason for the increase is that the Affordable Care Act of 2010 supports models that focus on care coordination. One of these models is the accountable care organization (ACO) (discussed earlier), which increased use of case management (Arnold, 2022). **Case Management** is "a collaborative process of assessment, planning, facilitation, care coordination, evaluation and advocacy for options and

United States Department of Health and Human Services (HHS), "Statement by HHS Secretary Xavier Becerra on Senate Passage of the Inflation Reduction Act," https://www.hhs.gov/about/news/2022/08/07/statement-by-hhs-secretary-xavier-becerra-on-senate-passage-of-the-inflation-reduction-act.html, 2022.

services to meet an individual's and family's comprehensive health needs through communication and available resources to Triple Aim: improve patient care, reduce costs, and improve population health. Case manager services emphasize wellness and autonomy by using advocacy, communication, education, identification of service resources, and service facilitation (CMSA, 2021). Case managers may be registered nurses, but this is not required; some may be social workers. It is not a specific profession as the role may be held by people from several different professions, but all case managers regardless of their profession require expertise in collaboration, coordination, and communication (Finkelman, 2011; 2021). Case managers may work in clinics, health departments, home healthcare agencies, long-term case sites, and hospitals.

Rehabilitation Services

Rehabilitation services may be found in ambulatory care centers, public health sites, homes, and long-term care settings. These services may be required after hospital discharge or for patients in the community who may not have been hospitalized. They offer support and focus on returning the patient to as positive functioning as possible and may include physical and psychological interventions such as physical therapy, occupational therapy, speech-language therapy, and mental health rehabilitation services. A variety of healthcare professionals provide these services, including physical therapists, occupational therapists, speech therapists, and psychologists.

Faith-Community Nursing

Faith-community nursing or parish nursing is found in some communities. These nurses are associated with a faith-based organization. They provide some health services to congregants focused on health promotion, chronic illness management, and safety or injury prevention (such as health education, referrals for further health care, guidance in the effective use of the healthcare system, support groups, and end-of-life support and guidance). The American Nurses Association has published standards for this specialty and describes it as "a nursing practice specialty that focuses on the intentional care of the spirit, the promotion of an integrative model of health, and the prevention and minimization of illness within the context of a faith community" (ANA, 2017). Registered nurses can be certified in this practice area.

The Federal Emergency Management Agency (FEMA), which is part of the Department of Homeland Security (DHS), recognizes the need to collaborate with faith-based organizations to better plan for emergencies and utilize these resources to assist in community response during public health emergencies (FEMA, 2018). **Figure 7** describes a seven-step engagement process that these organizations should take to prepare for emergencies and their responses. This initiative indicates that the federal government recognizes faith-based organizations as important stakeholders in all aspects of public and community health.

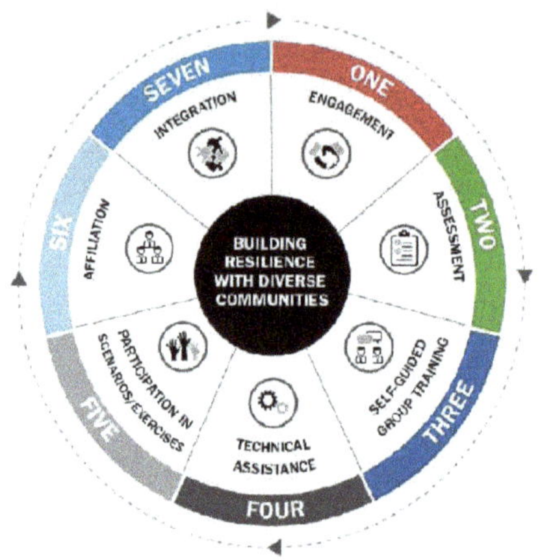

Figure 7. Seven-Step Engagement Process

Forensic Nursing Services

Forensic nursing is not a specialty that most in nursing consider or even know exists. It is an important part of public health settings that provide services to those who are in incarcerated or have other judicial problems. Correctional forensic nurses provide health care to those incarcerated in the criminal justice system (jails, prisons, and juvenile detention centers). Jails are managed by cities and counties. Prisons are managed by state or federal government. Juvenile detention centers are varied and can hold both pretrial and sentenced youth (IAFN, 2022a). These healthcare services include screening and monitoring, chronic care management, medication administration, and episodic sick call. Correctional facilities are part of many communities and may be local, state, or federal.

A specialized forensic nursing role is that of the sexual assault nurse examiner (SANE) (IAFN, 2022b). A registered nurse who wants to be a SANE must complete special training and may be certified in this nursing practice specialty. These services are managed through communities and are associated with a hospital, community program, or law enforcement. This is critical public health care, and it has ramifications for the judicial system. These nurses work directly with victims to provide support, assess health status, collect evidence, and refer victims for additional care and support. A SANE also may give testimony when cases go to trial.

Communities need to assess their services for sexual assault and provide services such as rape crisis centers and emergency helplines. Domestic abuse of all types also needs to be included in the assessment and provision of health services and emotional support. Public health departments may also provide shelters (for all genders and ages) for those in need, and within the shelters staff may provide healthcare services, which should include consideration of mental health and substance use. The CDC identifies intimate partner violence (IPV) as a public health problem (CDC, 2022c). It includes physical violence, sexual violence, stalking, and psychological aggression, which can include verbal or nonverbal communication with intent to harm or threaten. IVP impacts health and socioeconomic status. It is a serious problem that the CDC and other experts consider a preventable, but this requires assessment and active public health interventions. The following information provides an overview of the extent of the problem (CDC, 2022c):

- About 1 in 4 women and nearly 1 in 10 men have experienced sexual violence, physical violence, and/or stalking by an intimate partner during their lifetimes and reported some form of IPV-related impact.
- Over 43 million women and 38 million men have experienced psychological aggression by an intimate partner in their lifetimes.

Community Violence

Review the information on intimate partner violence at the site below. Consider how you might apply this information if your community assesses that there is an increase in intimate partner violence.

Website: https://www.cdc.gov/violenceprevention/intimatepartnerviolence/fastfact.html

Digital Health Services (Telehealth and Telemedicine)

Digital health services are increasing and are now part of public and community health services. They are either connected to other services or stand alone and use a variety of healthcare providers. These services include the use of various methods to provide and/or monitor health such as mobile health (mHealth), health information technology (HIT), wearable devices, telehealth and telemedicine, and personalized medicine. Telehealth has a broader definition than telemedicine, focusing on remote or digital healthcare that does not always involve clinical services. It may include use of videoconferencing, transmission of still images, e-health including patient portals, remote monitoring of vital signs, continuing professional healthcare education (e.g., medical, nursing, pharmacy) and nursing call centers. Telemedicine is a type of digital health which medical information is exchanged from one site to another via electronic communications and interventions may be provided. It is not considered a separate medical specialty and can be used by many healthcare providers.

The use of digital health, both telehealth and telemedicine, expanded during the COVID-19 pandemic and was useful for many patients. One study noted that "billing for remote patient monitoring increased more than fourfold during the first year of the COVID-19 pandemic. Most of this growth was driven by a small number of primary care providers. Among the patients of these providers with a high volume of remote patient monitoring, we did not observe substantial targeting of remote patient monitoring to people with greater disease burden or worse disease control" (Tang et al., 2022). However, despite this expansion, for example in Medicare telehealth utilization, there were disparities in use between Black and rural Medicare enrollees and White and urban enrollees (Pitsor, 2022). An example of a barrier to health services is the estimate by the Federal Communications Commission that as of 2019 at least 14.5 million people in the United States had insufficient broadband speeds, representing a major telehealth barrier. Limited access to computers and smartphones are also barriers. The expansion in this area of health care proved challenging due to these issues, and further use and development of new services need to consider these challenges to ensure access and health equity.

Public and Community Health Services' Relationship to Social Determinants of Health and Health Equity and Disparity

Public and community health provides comprehensive accessible services to a community or a population to ensure health needs are met. To be effective, services need to examine social determinants of health (SDOH) that affect the community and individuals and seek to prevent or reduce health disparities while supporting health equity. This requires increased emphasis on advocacy and policy development, with the goal of ensuring a healthy community. The following content examines this perspective.

Social Determinants of Health, Health Equity, and Disparities

The HHS is focusing more on ensuring equitable health outcomes, and this requires better coordination of health and human services and recognition of critical factors that impact health and social needs. There is diversity in communities, with differences in population characteristics such as gender, religion, ethnicity, and age, among others. Diversity needs to be assessed and recognized in planning and providing public and community services. It also impacts **health disparities**, which are a concern. These are "preventable differences in the burden of disease, injury, violence, or in opportunities to achieve optimal health experienced by socially disadvantaged racial, ethnic, and other population groups, and communities. Health disparities exist in all age groups, including older adults" (CDC, 2017).

The **social determinants of health** are "the conditions in the environments where people are born, live, learn, work, play, worship, and age that affect a wide range of health, functioning, and quality-of-life outcomes and risks" (ODPHP, 2020b). These factors are organized into five domains and have become a central part of public health and its services. They have a direct and significant impact on health outcomes. See **Figure 8**.

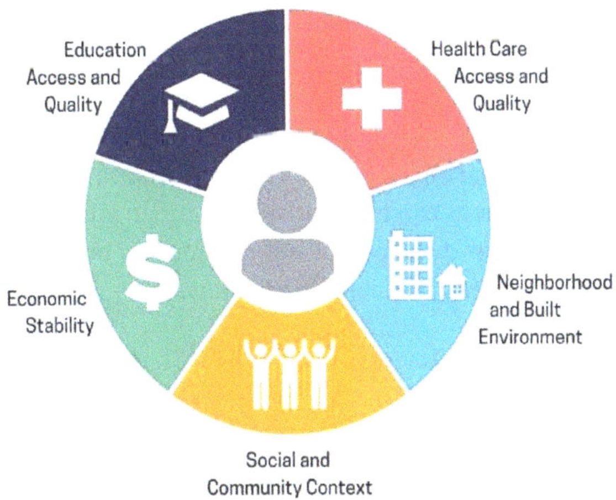

Figure 8. Social Determinants of Health

CDC, "Health Disparities," https://www.cdc.gov/aging/disparities/index.htm, 2017.

Why are the SDOH important? "It is estimated that clinical care accounts for only 20% of the county-level variation in health outcomes, while SDOH account for as much as 50% and are a major driver of health disparities" (Office of the Assistant Secretary for Planning and Evaluation, 2022). These factors are associated with **health equity**, which is achieved when

> all members of society enjoy a fair and just opportunity to be as healthy as possible. Public health policies and programs centered around the specific needs of communities can promote health equity. The HHS and its agencies such as the CDC are committed to understanding and appropriately addressing the needs of all populations, according to specific cultural, linguistic, and environmental factors. By ensuring health equity is integrated across all public health efforts, all communities will be stronger, safer, healthier, and more resilient. (CDC, 2022b)

Social Determinants of Health

Review the updates on SDOH. Select one of the SDOH domains that interests you. What can you learn about its status?

Website: https://health.gov/news/202208/weve-updated-healthy-people-2030-sdoh-literature-summaries?source=govdelivery&utm_medium=email&utm_source=govdelivery

Populations Experiencing Health Disparities

Vulnerable populations are populations at greater risk of experiencing health and social disparities due to social and economic factors such as SDOH. These populations can be found in both urban and rural areas. This section describes some of the public and community health services that can promote health equity for these populations.

Populations with Chronic Health Problems

People with chronic health problems require public and community health services. U.S. data on chronic disease or conditions indicates that 6 in 10 Americans have at least one chronic disease (NCCDPHP, 2022a). Many of the settings and services previously discussed apply to this population, for example, clinics, home health care, rehabilitation, and long-term care. People with chronic diseases are diverse, may vary in age and include children, and may have more than one chronic disease. They require healthcare guidance, coordination, and health education, along with interventions; access to medications and medical supplies; ongoing assessment to determine when needs change and services need to be altered, and so on. The CDC recognizes the need to address these problems through its National Center for Chronic Disease Prevention and Health Promotion. See **Figure 9**.

CHRONIC DISEASES IN AMERICA

6 IN 10
Adults in the US have a **chronic disease**

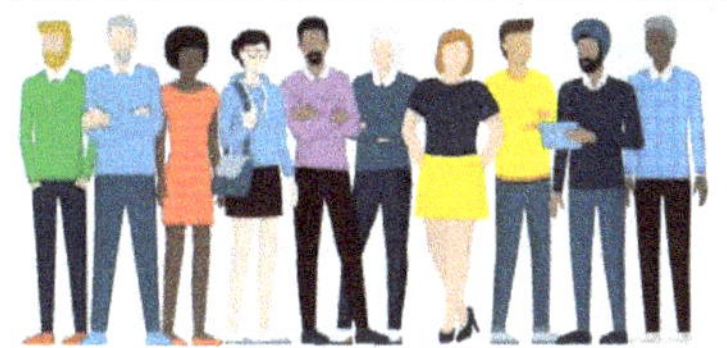

4 IN 10
Adults in the US have **two or more**

THE LEADING CAUSES OF DEATH AND DISABILITY
and Leading Drivers of the Nation's **$4.1 Trillion** in Annual Health Care Costs

Figure 9. Chronic Diseases in America

People with Disabilities

People with disabilities have many needs in communities and may have financial problems that limit access to health care and other social and economic concerns. Public health should consider the impact of payment for these health services. Medicaid expansion associated with the Affordable Care Act has led to an improvement in full-year insurance coverage for many, for example, by reducing out-of-pocket spending for adults with disabilities who are now eligible for Medicaid (Creedon et al., 2022). This improvement includes preventive care and some primary care measures. Some of the services that people with disabilities may need are routine health care/primary care; care for specific disabilities that may include specialists; assistive equipment such as walkers or wheelchairs; physical therapy, which is provided in the community or at home; special education; and support in coping with disabilities. These services may be offered in a variety of public health settings, and for many people disabilities represent long-term needs. Social services are also often required for people with disabilities, for example, assistance with financial concerns, housing, access to food, transportation, employment options, and other services.

Children and Teens

Well-childcare has been part of pediatric primary care for many years. These services are recommended for all children and offered in a variety of settings such as pediatrician's and nurse practitioner's practices, clinics, and public health departments. A recent study noted that there are problems with health equity leading to disparities in meeting the health recommendations of regular well-childcare visits to ensure the long-term health of children. Reduction in well-childcare has long-term consequences for children's and adolescents' health and can impact health in adulthood. Abdus and Selden (2022) find that, between 2006 and 2007 and 2016 and 2017, well-child visit adherence rose from 47.9% to 62.3%. However, "among uninsured children in 2016 and 2017, adherence was only half the national average, and more than 20 percentage points separated the highest- and lowest-adherence geographic regions of the nation. The disparity between White non-Hispanic and Black non-Hispanic children widened during the period." Well-child checks are important in identifying health concerns, monitoring growth and development, assessing hearing and eyesight, administering and monitoring immunizations, and offering parents or caregivers opportunities to ask questions and receive health education about their children and parenting. This service is also important in identifying mental health concerns and issues such as abuse.

It is important to note that from 2019–2021 more children under the age of 19 became covered by health insurance than in the past (Mykyta et al., 2022). This resulted in 475,000 fewer children without coverage compared to the years before 2019, a critical factor in increasing health equity and reducing health disparities in children. The two major government health insurance programs that have made a difference are Medicaid and the Children's Health Insurance Program (CHIP). Medicaid provides coverage for children and adults with incomes below certain levels. CHIP provides health insurance for children in families with income too high to qualify for Medicaid but that typically cannot afford private health insurance. During the COVID-19 pandemic funding was expanded to ensure coverage for more children who needed it.

Families

Families are connected to all health settings and are a critical part of public and community health. Communities need to assess the health of families and identify both health and social needs. School health is involved in family health as nurses work with children and their parents. School health practitioners can often identify families in need. Some clinics focus on family health. They provide primary care services are for children of all ages and adults (e.g., parents). Family health centers are good sites to offer wraparound services so that multiple needs can be addressed at one site, for example, social services, access to food sources, legal help, and so on. Communities with diverse populations need to consider factors such as language and culture as they provide family health services.

Pregnant Women

> In the United States of America, in the 21st century, being pregnant and giving birth should not carry such great risk. And yet, before, during, and after childbirth, women in our country are dying at a higher rate from pregnancy-related causes than in any other developed nation. For certain women, the risk is much higher. Regardless of income or education level, Black women are three times as likely to die from pregnancy-related complications. Native American women are more than twice as likely to die. And women who live in rural America—where there are many maternal care deserts—are about 60 percent more likely to die. These outcomes are largely due to systemic inequities, which create significant disparities in how women experience the healthcare system that can often be a matter of life and death. (White House, 2022, p. 1)

To address these concerns the White House under the Biden administration plans on "cutting the rates of maternal mortality and morbidity, reducing the disparities in maternal health outcomes, and improving the overall experience of pregnancy, birth, and postpartum for people across the country" (White House, 2022, p. 3). This initiative is also connected with other initiatives to advance health equity and reduce disparities for communities experiencing health disparities (HHS Press Office, 2022b). Since most maternal child services take place in the community, this blueprint applies to community health services and to public health provided in ambulatory care, health departments, and through social services. In addition, communities need to expand health education for women before, during, and after pregnancy. Women need nutrition guidance, preparation for delivery and postpartum, guidance on care of newborns, assessment during postpartum (for example, for postpartum depression), and general health services including pharmacy access. Access is important along with the recognition that women may need support such as childcare during appointments. Transportation is also an important factor in ensuring access to services, such as cost, parking, schedule, and so on. To improve care and access to this population the HHS, through its agency HRSA, increased funding to support community-based doulas, trained staff who support women during pregnancy and during postpartum, increase the use of home visits for parents and infants, support early childhood needs, and increase interventions in communities to decrease maternal mortality (HRSA, 2022c). Funding also supports staff training to reduce health disparities during pregnancy and postpartum.

An example of a federal program that supports pregnant women and families is the Maternal, Infant, and Early Childhood Home Visiting (MIECHV) Program. This service is offered through HRSA for families living in communities that are economically and experience barriers to achieving positive maternal and child health outcomes. "Families choose to participate in home visiting programs, and partner with health, social service, and child development professionals to set and achieve goals that improve their health and well-being" (HRSA, 2022c). The goals of the MIECHV Program are to

- improve maternal and child health
- prevent child abuse and neglect
- reduce crime and domestic violence
- increase family education level and earning potential
- promote children's development and readiness to participate in school
- connect families to needed community resources and supports

This type of service supports health and social needs for families, including both adults and children, and requires engagement from communities, healthcare providers and organizations, and social services.

Older Adults

An age-friendly health system focuses on evidence-based practice, causes no harm, and emphasizes what matters to older adults and their family caregivers (IHI, 2022a; 2022b). This type of system might apply the *4M* framework, which focuses on (1) what *m*atters, (2) *m*obility, (3) *m*entation, and (4) *m*edications. This topic has become more important as the older population increases, and this has led to the development of more resources to better ensure quality care. A resource on the 4M framework, developed by the John A. Hartford Foundation (JAHF) and the Institute for Health Improvement (IHI), is *Age Friendly Health Systems: A Guide to Using the 4Ms While Caring for Older Adults* (2022). The rural health site also emphasizes the need for age-friendly communities, supporting older adults who live in the community (RHI Hub, 2019).

The 4M Framework for an Age-Friendly System

View a description of the 4M framework at the following link. What is your view of this framework?

Website: https://www.youtube.com/watch?v=E2rUnWNjG54

The results of a study conducted by the National Cancer Institute and National Institutes of Health noted that leisure time activities have a positive impact on older adult health status, which has implications for communities (NIH, 2022b). Examples of the activities identified in this research are walking, jogging, swimming laps, playing tennis, and other similar activities for exercise. Exercise may lower mortality for any cause, particularly cardiovascular disease and cancer. What does this mean for public health in communities? Providing easy and safe access to exercise activities for older adults is important. This might include ensuring safe areas for walking and jogging in public parks, providing access to water and shade, and so on. In addition, public health facilities should encourage older adults to participate in exercise by providing information on its value and access.

A problem found in many communities is elder abuse, which is a form of interpersonal violence and relates to SDOH in the older adult. "Elder abuse is defined as an intentional act or failure to act by a caregiver or another person in a relationship involving an expectation of trust that causes or creates a risk of harm to an older adult (typically defined as age 60 years and older), and comprises 5 subtypes: physical abuse, sexual abuse, psychological abuse, caregiver neglect, and financial exploitation and fraud" (Mao, 2022). This abuse negatively impacts health outcomes and should be assessed and addressed by community healthcare providers. Often older adults do not report this abuse, so it is important that it is considered in assessment when older adults receive health and social services. The following are examples of healthcare provider interventions that are important with this population (Mao, 2022):

- Talk to patients and be aware of the red flags of elder abuse.
- Document abuse.
- Refer patients for assistance as need (for example, to Adult Protective Services) or get information from the Elder Justice website (https://www.justice.gov/elderjustice).

Elder Abuse

To learn more about elder abuse and the red flags indicating possible abuse, review the website below. Are you surprised by this information? If so, what surprised you and why? How might you use this information as a public health provider?

Website: https://ncea.acl.gov/NCEA/media/docs/Red-Flags-of-Elder-Abuse-English.pdf

Housing alternatives supporting aging in place, or continuing to live in the home one chooses, include several options. Independent living is any type of residential setting in which people live independently.

- *Active adult communities and independent living communities:* Residents have their own living space and access to many services—meals, housekeeping, activities, exercise, health care, and so on.
- *Assisted living residence:* Residents may live in their own space, but they require some assistance with tasks such as personal care, housekeeping, and support for daily healthcare needs. This is often viewed as a transition to more intensive care provided by a nursing home environment.
- *Nursing homes:* Settings that provide 24/7 care as need (discussed earlier in this content).

There are now communities that offer all these levels of service in one place, with residents transitioning from one level to another as needs change.

LGBTQ+ Population

This population has varying health needs and may require support. Schools may be one source of assistance and referral. Communities may also offer clinics to address the health needs of the LGBTQ+ community and should engage this population in assessing their needs and evaluating outcomes. They also may need social services or mental health and substance use interventions.

Racial and Ethnic Minorities and People Experiencing Economic Disadvantages

These populations are at risk for health disparities and poor health outcomes. Communities need to determine the status of these populations on a regular basis, recognizing that they have complex needs that impact health and access to health services. Social services in these communities are involved in ensuring multiple needs are met related to health, safe and sufficient housing, transportation, employment, education, family stress and support, safety, nutrition and access to food, crime and violence, and many other factors related to SDOH and health equity. All types of health services should provide effective assessment and access to services. For example, health clinics and other settings need to consider on-site access to social services, convenient hours of operation (since many people work different hours), transportation access, and so on. Wraparound services are also important to these populations to address multiple needs such as social services, access to food sources, legal services more effectively at one site, for example.

People Experiencing Homelessness

This population needs accessible healthcare services. Many people who have no housing or temporary housing have chronic illnesses. Living in this type of situation is not conducive to maintaining healthy habits and meeting medical needs for complex health problems and may lead to more health problems. Diet, exercise, environment, lack of opportunity to keep clean, poor sleep, stress, weather (heat and cold), and safety issues all impact the health of people experiencing homelessness and people in temporary housing. Some communities offer health services in areas where homeless people may be found, and this is an effective approach to accessibility. Often, this population does not trust systems such as the local health system due to negative prior experiences. Clinics and urgent care sites may be good sources of care, but staff need to be aware of complex needs, use effective nonthreatening communication, support follow-up methods, and work with services that provide housing and social services for this population.

Migrants, Refugees, and Immigrants

Migrant workers are typically found in rural areas and work in agriculture. Rural sources of public health need to be aware of this population and include them in local services, reaching out to them so that they know they can receive care. The same is true for refugees and immigrants, who can be found in both urban and rural areas. Language may be a critical factor in meeting health needs along with culture and religious differences. All these factors should be considered when sharing information about services and during the healthcare process. This population may need routine primary care, immunizations, management of chronic illnesses, and assistance with accidents and injuries.

Rural Populations

Recognizing the need to improve rural and tribal health services, funding of nearly $60 million was approved as part of the American Rescue Plan in August 2022. This initiative addresses the needs of a fifth of the U.S. population to (HHS Press Office, 2022f) and has the following goals:

- Reduce morbidity and mortality due to substance use disorders, such as training first responders in coping with opioid overdoses.
- Increase quality and operational improvements.
- Support rural hospitals that provide services for people with Medicare insurance.
- Develop state networks on rural health that link communities with state, federal, and non-profit resources with the goal of long-term solutions to improve rural health.

- Support medical training in rural health practice settings.
- Improve health care provision in tribal communities experiencing barriers such as remote locations.
- Improve telehealth, which is an important method for expanding access to care and improving health equity, especially for rural communities and communities that are medically underserved.
- Improve services for maternal health in rural areas through the Rural Maternity and Obstetrics Management Strategies (RMOMS) program.

In addition to these needs and services, there is also additional funding available to assist rural healthcare providers with expenses and lost revenues experienced during the COVID-19 pandemic. Rural areas were particularly hard hit by the pandemic, and this impacts their current public health needs and ability to respond to community needs. A recent HRSA report to Congress discussed improving access to care in underserved rural communities, and made the following recommendations (National Health Service Corps, 2022):

- Incorporate longitudinal clinical training in rural primary health.
- Integrate oral and behavioral health in primary health.
- Enhance the capacity of telehealth.
- Support interprofessional team-based education and practice in maternal-infant care.

This report identifies primary care health disparities between rural and urban areas that should be examined and improved. One of the barriers to improvement is the need for more healthcare provider training and practice settings. The above recommendations were made to address these disparities.

Medicare providers in rural areas can apply to be certified as rural health clinics (RHCs) (RHI Hub, 2021). Rural health clinics may be confused with Federally Qualified Health Centers (FQHCs). Exhibit 1 compares the two models, both of which can provide public and community health in rural areas.

As noted earlier, accountable care organizations are increasing, and this also impacts rural health. In a study of ACOs in rural areas, in addition to recognition of greater use, it was noted that ACOs are expanding their preventive and chronic disease management services, which are both important in rural areas (Bagwell, Bushy, & Ortiz, 2017). The study also indicated that information technology needs to improve to better integrate clinical and financial data in ACOs. Communities are recognizing the value of this type of setting and its services. ACOs provide additional sources for care in these areas where there is a shortage of services.

Exhibit 1. Differences Between RHCs and FQHCs

Rural Health Clinics	Federally Qualified Health Centers
For-profit or non-profit	Non-profit or public facility
May be limited to a specific type of primary care practice (e.g., OB-GYN, pediatrics)	Required to provide care for all age groups
Not required to have a board of directors	Required to have a board of directors—at least 51% must be patients of the health center
No minimum service requirements	Minimum services required include maternity and prenatal care, preventive care, behavioral health, dental health, emergency care, and pharmaceutical services
Not required to charge based on a sliding fee scale	Required to treat all residents in their service area with charges based on a sliding fee scale
Not required to provide a minimum of hours or emergency coverage	Required to be open 32.5 hours a week for Federal Tort Claims Act (FTCA) coverage of licensed or certified healthcare providers. Must provide emergency service after business hours either on site or by arrangement with another healthcare provider
Required to conduct a biennial program evaluation regarding quality improvement	Required to have ongoing quality assurance program
Must be located in a Health Professional Shortage Area, Medically Underserved Area, or governor-designated and secretary-certified shortage area. May retain RHC status if designation of service area changes	Must be located in an area that is underserved or experiencing a shortage of healthcare providers
RHCs must be in non-urbanized areas	FQHCs may operate in both non-urbanized and urbanized areas
Required to submit an annual cost report; however, auditing of financial reports is not required	Required to submit an annual cost report and audited financial report

Source: Rural Health Information Hub (RHI Hub). (2021, April 22). Rural health clinics (RHCs). *Human Resources and Services Administration (HRSA). https://www.ruralhealthinfo.org/topics/rural-health-clinics*

Persons Who Experience Mental Health Problems

Community mental health centers and community-based sites that include mental health care as one of their services are important in public health. In addition, all public health services should be aware of signs and symptoms of mental health problems, assess for these problems, and provide services or referrals for individuals of all ages, families, and couples. These health needs have increased with the recent COVID-19 pandemic. For example, the American Academy of Pediatrics (AAP), American Academy of Child and Adolescent Psychiatry, and Children's Hospital Association declared a national emergency in child and adolescent mental health (AAP, 2021). This is also associated with the Biden Administration's declaration about mental health. Other service needs for this population are mental health or behavioral health crisis centers and suicide hotlines. Communities need to do more to prevent mental health problems, such as offering stress management resources in the community, schools, and even businesses. There has been an increasing problem with polypharmacy for the treatment of mental health problems, particularly with children and teens. Healthcare providers in communities need to evaluate and monitor the use of medications carefully. Law enforcement should also be trained to recognize and respond appropriately to stress and mental health problems they may encounter in the community and know how to connect those in need with effective care. Increasing violence is often associated with mental health problems. An example is domestic abuse, which is mentioned in the forensic nursing section. Law enforcement is often involved in these incidents and should have resources to guide those involved to assistance and supportive services.

A barrier to improving mental health services is the lack of healthcare providers with this expertise. The typical provider has traditionally been a psychiatrist, but there is a nationwide shortage of psychiatrists. Other providers are needed, and an example is the increasing use of psychiatric mental health nurse practitioners (PMHNPs). This new group of providers can increase services and reach populations that need active treatment. In a study that examined this expansion and its outcomes, it is noted that

> from 2011 to 2019, the number of PMHNPs treating Medicare beneficiaries grew 162 percent, compared with a 6 percent relative decrease in the number of psychiatrists doing so. During the same period, total annual mental health office visits per 100 beneficiaries decreased 11.5 percent from 27.4 to 24.2, the net result of a 29.0 percent drop in psychiatrist visits being offset by a 111.3 percent increase in nurse practitioner visits. The proportion of all mental health prescriber visits provided

by PMHNPs increased from 12.5 percent to 29.8 percent during 2011–19, exceeding 50 percent in rural, full-scope-of-practice regions. PMHNPs are a rapidly growing workforce that may be instrumental in improving mental health care access. (Cai et al., 2022)

Suicide Hotlines

Suicide hotlines have been used for many years, but there are communities that lack effective services and support. Some changes are in process. Review the following discussion. Identify the problems and the populations at greater risk. What needs to be done to improve access to suicide hotlines?

Website: https://khn.org/news/article/988-mental-health-suicide-prevention-hotline-network-rural-areas-service-shortages/?utm_campaign=KHN%3A%20Daily%20Health%20Policy%20Report&utm_medium=email&_hsmi=221104456&_hsenc=p2ANqtz--FLU6tcn03ZOBKL-ehV7pbaYG7IA4hviKmbtyAqC9DDzB2DVjKkecGJzV1MIcYRjD9pUCZXmfupq3VF40QabtMr0Y6WQ&utm_content=221104456&utm_source=hs_email

The WHO published an extensive report on global mental health problems (2022b). The report identifies four healthcare roles required to support effective mental health for all: (1) promote mental health, (2) prevent mental health problems, (3) provide care, and (4) work in partnership and support related initiatives. There are many factors that influence mental health status that should be recognized in public health services, including individual psychological and biological factors; family and community factors; and structural factors such as environment, infrastructure, social stability, access to services, and basic needs, and include risks such as disease, conflict, discrimination, disparities, and social injustice. Public and community health services need to develop and support resilience by considering protective factors, such as family, positive parenting, good working environments, safe neighborhoods, education, basic needs for nutrition and housing being met, and so on. Economic and social inequalities can lead to mental health problems or make these problems worse. Public health emergencies such as a disaster or an epidemic/pandemic increase stress for individuals, populations, and communities. This impacts mental health during crises and can have long-term impacts. People experience anxiety, depression, fear, and more. They turn to public sources for support, but if they think they are not receiving clear and accurate information, then anxiety and distrust in the community increases and negatively impacts their mental health. Other situations that impact mental health globally are conflicts and climate change, which has caused major crises for many due to high temperatures, storms, floods, and fires. The WHO report identifies the following as global concerns (2022b, p. 36):

- "In all countries, mental disorders are highly prevalent and largely undertreated.
- Mental disorders are the leading cause of years lived with disability, and suicide remains a major cause of death globally.
- The economic consequences of mental health conditions are enormous, with productivity losses significantly outstripping the direct costs of care.
- Mental health systems all over the world are marked by major gaps in governance, resources, [and] services information and technologies for mental health.
- Several factors stop people from seeking help for mental health conditions, including limited access to quality services, low levels of health literacy about mental health, and pervasive stigma."

Persons Who Experience Substance Use Disorder

Community-based services for substance use are important. This is a growing need across the United States. Some communities are experiencing extreme crisis with opioid use and other substances leading to long-term health problems and death. Alcohol use is also a problem. Substance use may lead to other community problems such as traffic accidents, violence and domestic abuse, suicide and overdoses, family problems and divorce, crime, law enforcement issues, difficulties with school (not attending, unable to do coursework), bullying, erratic employment, inability to work, loss of housing, financial problems, and so on. All public health services should be alert to the signs and symptoms of this problem and intervene in an effective manner. This requires an interprofessional approach that includes community members, healthcare providers and organizations, social services, schools, faith-community organizations, law enforcement, and government.

Local, State, and Federal Government Involvement in Public and Community Health Services

Effective public and community health services are associated with local, state, and federal government activities. Collaboration, coordination, and communication among all levels of government are critical, along with joint planning, implementation, and evaluation of outcomes. Communities at all levels should be involved in surveillance, data collection and analysis, sharing information, and identifying problems and strategies to address them. This section discusses examples of government activities.

Local, State, and Federal Government

Local and state health departments are responsible for public health in their communities. They collaborate with the federal government through the U.S. Department of Health and Human Services and its many agencies. All levels of government make laws and regulations that relate to public and community health services and provide some funding for these activities. Some of the funding is shared, for example, between local and state or state and federal agencies. State and federal government health departments provide resources; conduct public health research; collect data to provide information about needs, strategies, and outcomes; and offer health programs and services.

The U.S. Public Health Service (USPHS) is an important federal public health resource. The USPHS "works on the front lines of public health ... medical, health and engineering professionals fight disease, conduct research, and care for patients in underserved communities across the nation and throughout the world, to protect, promote, and advance the health and safety of the nation" (USPHS, 2022). Members of this uniformed services branch work at the CDC, FDA, NIH, Indian Health Services, the Federal Bureau of Prisons, and the Department of Defense. Professionals involved include physicians, nurses, dentists, pharmacists, therapists, dieticians, veterinarians, scientists, and engineers. The USPHS also provides health services related to environmental health issues.

Examples of Major Population Policies, Programs, and Interventions

The following content describes population policies, programs, and interventions that support public and community health services.

Office of Disease Prevention and Health Promotion

The Office of Disease Prevention and Health Promotion (ODPHP) "encourages all Americans to lead healthy and active lives. We accomplish this by establishing and promoting national public health priorities; translating science into policy, guidance, and tools; and working to improve health literacy and equitable access to clear and actionable health information" (ODPHP, 2022b). Health promotion and **disease prevention** are critical elements of public health. The major ODPHP initiatives are Healthy People, Healthy Aging, and Health Literacy. In addition, the ODPHP offers events and strategies to address changing needs, for example, August 2022 was declared National Immunization Awareness Month to share information with the public about the need for immunizations and the upcoming flu season (ODPHP, 2022a).

Related to the ODPHP activities is the need for strategic planning to ensure disease prevention and health promotion. The Affordable Care Act of 2010 included recommendations to create the National Prevention Council to guide the nation's prevention strategy and partner with the Office of the Surgeon General in meeting this goal. Integrating evidence-based recommendations for the leading causes of disability and death is part of this initiative. The following are the four strategic directions and the priorities (NIH, 2014):

1. healthy and safe community environments
2. clinical and community preventive services
3. empowered people
4. elimination of health disparities

The prevention priorities are:

- tobacco-free living
- preventing drug abuse and excessive alcohol use
- healthy eating
- active living
- injury- and violence-free living
- reproductive and sexual health
- mental and emotional well-being

Consumer Assessment of Healthcare Providers and Systems (CAHPS®)

The Consumer Assessment of Healthcare Providers and Systems (CAHPS®) developed the Home and Community-Based Services Survey and works with the AHRQ to implement the survey (AHRQ, 2022b). The purpose of the survey is to assess adult Medicaid beneficiaries' experience with long-term care. The AHRQ administers the survey, with data collected through in-person or telephone interviews. The focus is on evaluating some of the programs that provide services for adults with disabilities, including the frail elderly and people with physical disabilities, developmental or intellectual disabilities, acquired brain injury, or severe mental illness. The questions addressed in the survey include content related to the following (AHRQ, 2022b):

National Institutes of Health (NIH), "The National Prevention Strategy: Prioritizing Prevention to Improve the Nation's Health," https://prevention.nih.gov/education-training/methods-mind-gap/national-prevention-strategy-prioritizing-prevention-improve-nations-health, 2020.

- getting needed services
- communication with providers
- access to case managers
- choice of services
- medical transportation
- personal safety
- community inclusion and empowerment

The database associated with this survey provides information about services provided by state Medicaid agencies and contracted managed care organizations. The database is used to obtain the following information (AHRQ, 2022b):

- Raise general awareness about the home and community-based care experience.
- Diagnose and assess the current status of patient experiences and programs.
- Identify strengths and opportunities for patient experience improvement.
- Examine trends in home and community-based patient experience over time.
- Evaluate the impact of patient experience improvement initiatives and interventions.

Healthy People 2030

Healthy People 2030 collects and analyzes evaluation data for many health and healthcare delivery topics and identifies goals and objectives that are used in measurement. The goals focus on many areas of healthcare concern such as vulnerable populations, specific health problems, and topics related to public health services. These goals recognize that communities have an impact on health and well-being; preventive services should be provided by communities; schools are sources of public health services; healthy and safe home environments are important to individual, family, and community health; and workplaces offer opportunities to better ensure public health and should be safe environments. The box below offers more information about these goals and related objectives. **Appendix A** provides more information about Healthy People 2030.

National Healthcare Quality and Disparities Report

The *National Healthcare Quality and Disparities Report* provides annual data on healthcare quality and disparities. Its measures focus on access to care, affordable care, care coordination, effective treatment, healthy living, patient safety, and person-centered care (AHRQ, 2022c). Information on disparities considers race and ethnicity, income, and other SDOH. This information is useful in assessing public health services and identifying needs and changes that may be required to meet Health People 2030 goals and improve public health in a variety of settings.

Healthy People: Public and Community Health Goals

Healthy People 2030 has several goals related to public and community health services and the content in this guide. Review the status of the objectives for each of the following goals at the links provided.

- **Goal: Promote health and safety in community settings.** https://health.gov/healthypeople/objectives-and-data/browse-objectives#settings-and-systems
- **Goal: Promote healthy and safe home environments.** https://health.gov/healthypeople/objectives-and-data/browse-objectives/housing-and-homes
- **Goal: Promote health, safety, and learning in school settings.** https://health.gov/healthypeople/objectives-and-data/browse-objectives/schools
- **Goal: Promote the health and safety of people at work.** https://health.gov/healthypeople/objectives-and-data/browse-objectives/workplace

Health Literacy

The Healthy People 2030 initiative is the first version of the Healthy People initiative that includes health literacy in its goals. The definition of health literacy was changed to include both personal and organizational perspectives and the recognition that improving health literacy is a significant challenge (Santana et al., 2021). The HHS recognizes that there are many stakeholders who need to be involved in ensuring effective health literacy, such as consumers, businesses, educators, government agencies, health insurers, community leaders, healthcare providers, the media, and other community organizations (nonprofit, faith-based, etc.). The two **health literacy** definitions are (CDC, 2022a):

- "Personal health literacy is the degree to which individuals can find, understand, and use information and services to inform health-related decisions and actions for themselves and others.
- Organizational health literacy is the degree to which organizations equitably enable individuals to find, understand, and use information and services to inform health-related decisions and actions for themselves and others."

CDC Population Health Initiatives

The CDC, through its Division on Population Health (DPH), collects, analyzes, and shares data about chronic diseases, risk factors, and outcomes. This information is important in assisting the DPH, all levels of government, and public and community health programs to apply data and analysis to develop prevention strategies for specific populations and settings. This can facilitate the development and use of innovative public health programs, prevention research, and the increased use of evidence-based practices in public and community health settings (NCCDPHP, 2022b). DPH is an important resource for public and community health and its many healthcare settings and services.

HRSA Special Initiatives for Vulnerable Populations

HRSA's strategic planning is concerned with operational-level planning and resource allocation. Its goals are the following (HRSA, 2021a):

1. Improve access to quality health services.
2. Foster a healthcare workforce able to address current and emerging needs.
3. Achieve health equity and enhance population health.
4. Optimize HRSA operations and strengthen program management.

HRSA is involved in providing public health resources to communicate the best health information to the public. Examples include poison control; women's healthy living guides; stopbullying.gov; and resources for women, infants, and children (HRSA, 2022a).

Healthcare providers and other staff are needed to ensure that healthcare services are accessible and effective. HRSA provides funding to support the healthcare workforce. A recent initiative provides $100 million to fund state run programs that support, recruit, and retain primary care clinicians who live and work in underserved communities. Some of the healthcare providers are part of the National Health Service Corps (NHSC), which "builds healthy communities by supporting qualified health care providers dedicated to working in areas of the United States with limited access to care" (HHS Press Office, 2021).

HRSA also offers resources for public and community health to ensure the safe transition of patients out of ambulatory care services (AHRQ, 2017). This is an example of how the federal government supports national public health and local and state health departments and their services. Care transition is a time of increased risk for error in providing services, and often this occurs due to ineffective communication, collaboration, and coordination. Transition post-hospitalization, such as what was experienced during the

COVID-19 pandemic, is an important issue for communities. What type of care transition model should a community consider and develop (Landor et al., 2020)? Nurse coordinators can be effective in collaborating with multidisciplinary teams and ensuring that at-risk patients are identified, establishing a first point of contact, connecting the patient to appropriate provider(s) in the community, and ensuring effective follow-up care. The patient is also connected to their regular primary care provider (PCP) or to a new PCP. Some patients may require home care, additional ambulatory care, or long-term care with more support.

Research and Public and Community Health Services

The National Institute of Nursing Research (NINR) strategic plan for 2022–2026 focuses on "five research areas (referred to as 'lenses'): health equity, social determinants of health, population and community health, prevention and health promotion, and systems and models of care" (NINR, 2022). **Figure 10** describes the NINR strategic plan. Evidence-based practice is a key component of nursing practice, and this includes public and community health. The NINR strategic plan supports evidence-based practice and the need for research to improve practices in all communities and for all populations.

An example of the impact that research results can have on public health is found in a recent National Institute of Health (NIH) study (NIH, 2022a). This

MISSION: Lead nursing research to solve pressing health challenges and inform practice and policy—optimizing health and advancing health equity into the future.

RESEARCH LENSES

Health Equity

Reduce and ultimately eliminate the systemic and structural inequities that place some at an unfair, unjust, and avoidable disadvantage in attaining their full health potential.

Social Determinants of Health

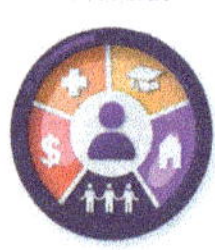

Identify effective approaches to improve health and quality of life by addressing the conditions in which people are born, live, learn, work, play, and age.

Population and Community Health

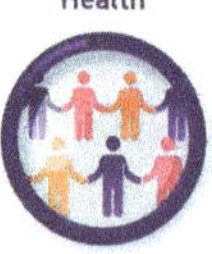

Address critical health challenges at a macro level that persistently affect groups of people with shared characteristics.

Prevention and Health Promotion

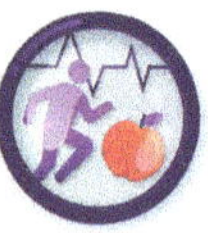

Prevent disease and promote health through the continuum of prevention—from primordial to tertiary.

Systems and Models of Care

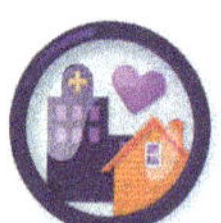

Address clinical, organizational, and policy challenges through new systems and models of care.

Figure 10. NINR 2022–2026 Strategic Plan

study examined cardiovascular deaths in the United States. The results note that mortality has decreased in the last two decades, but problems continue with health disparities and inequities. Factors that impact cardiovascular deaths are differences in race and ethnicity, geographic location, and access to care. These factors must be considered in public and community health to reduce the risk of a negative health outcome for vulnerable populations. Evidence-based interventions are required to make changes and improve. The study's literature review indicates that younger Black adults are an at-risk group but are often missed in identifying risk. Other at-risk populations noted in the study are women and people who are incarcerated. All of these groups should be receiving comprehensive health care. Communities need to consider multiple strategies to assess all populations, such as using innovative approaches to increase blood pressure screening and health education at nontraditional sites (e.g., hair salons and barbershops, schools, grocery stores, and faith-community buildings).

Summary

There is a greater need for nurses to work in primary care and for interprofessional collaboration, coordination, and communication. This content reviewed multiple public and community health settings and services. Healthcare profession education, including nursing education, needs to expand content and experiences for students so that they are prepared and this may increase interest in practicing in these types of settings. This content emphasizes that clinical experiences need to include primary care, care coordination and chronic disease management, prevention and health promotion, examination of the independent community-based primary care role, and the development of services in communities, among other health settings and roles. The expansion in practice includes "full-scope, autonomous, holistic nursing in primary care. However, more work is required to address role clarity, enhance nurses' understanding of what full-scope RN practice looks like, develop the business case for RN integration onto the primary care team, and advocate for policy changes that recognize RN contributions for service delivery and reimbursement" (Dolansky & Livsey, 2021, p. 80).

Discussion Questions

1. How does the public health framework relate to public health services? Provide two examples.
2. How might a clinic incorporate health equity in its services?

3. Select two of the public health services described in this content and describe how each service relates to one of the vulnerable populations identified.
4. If you are considering a position in public health, which of the healthcare settings discussed in the content interests you as a practice setting? Provide a rationale for your choice.
5. Why is it important to have effective collaboration, coordination, and communication in public health at the local, state, and federal levels of government?

References

Abdus, S., & Selden, T. (2022, August 22). Well-child visit adherence. *JAMA Pediatrics, 176*(11), 1143–1145. https://doi.org/10.1001/jamapediatrics.2022.2954

Agency for Healthcare Research and Quality (AHRQ). (2017). *Toolkit to engage high-risk patients in safe transitions across ambulatory care settings.* U.S. Department of Health and Human Services (HHS). https://www.ahrq.gov/hai/tools/ambulatory-care/safe-transitions.html

Agency for Healthcare Research and Quality (AHRQ). (2018, February). *Ambulatory care.* U.S. Department of Health and Human Services (HHS). https://www.ahrq.gov/patient-safety/settings/ambulatory/tools.html

Agency for Healthcare Research and Quality (AHRQ). (2022a, August). *Defining the PCMH.* U.S. Department of Health and Human Services (HHS). https://www.ahrq.gov/ncepcr/tools/pcmh/defining/index.html

Agency for Healthcare Research and Quality (AHRQ). (2022b, October). *CAHPS home and community based survey.* U.S. Department of Health and Human Services (HHS). https://www.ahrq.gov/cahps/surveys-guidance/hcbs/index.html

Agency for Healthcare Research and Quality (AHRQ). (2022c, October). *National healthcare quality and disparities reports.* U.S. Department of Health and Human Services (HHS). https://www.ahrq.gov/research/findings/nhqrdr/index.html

American Academy of Ambulatory Care Nursing (AAACN). (2017). *Scope and standards of practice for professional ambulatory care nursing.* Pitman, NJ: Author.

American Academy of Ambulatory Care Nursing (AAACN). (2018). *Scope and standards of practice for professional telehealth nursing* (6th ed.). Pitman, NJ: Author.

American Academy of Ambulatory Care Nursing (AAACN). (2022). *Defining characteristics.* https://www.aaacn.org/practice-resources/what-ambulatory-care-nursing/defining-characteristics

American Academy of Family Physicians (AAFP). (2022). *Retail clinics.* https://www.aafp.org/about/policies/all/retail-clinics.html

American Academy of Nursing (AAN). (2021). *Nurse-managed health centers: National nursing centers consortium & institute for nursing centers.* https://www.aannet.org/initiatives/edge-runners/profiles/edge-runners--nurse-managed-health-centers

American Academy of Pediatrics (AAP). (2021, October 19). *A declaration from the American Academy of Pediatrics, American Academy of Child and Adolescent Psychiatry and Children's Hospital Association.* https://www.aap.org/en/advocacy/child-and-adolescent-healthy-mental-development/aap-aacap-cha-declaration-of-a-national-emergency-in-child-and-adolescent-mental-health/

American Association of Occupational Health Nurses (AAOHN). (2022). *What is occupational & environmental health nursing?* https://www.aaohn.org/About/What-is-Occupational-and-Environmental-Health-Nursing

American Nurses Association (ANA). (2017). *Faith community nursing: Scope and standards of practice.*

American Nurses Association (ANA). (2022). *Public health nursing: Scope & standards of practice* (3rd. ed.).

American Public Health Association (APHA). (2021a). *What is public health?* https://www.apha.org/What-is-Public-Health

American Public Health Association (APHA). (2021b). *Community health workers.* https://www.apha.org/apha-communities/member-sections/community-health-workers

Arnold, S. (2022). Case management: An overview for nurses. *Nursing2022, 49*(9), 43–45.

Bagwell, M. T., Bushy, A., & Ortiz, J. (2017, January). Accountable care organization implementation experiences and rural participation. *Journal of Nursing Administration, 47*(1), 30–34.

Blumenthal, D., Collins, S. R., & Fowler, E. (2020, February 26). *The Affordable Care Act at 10 years: What's the effect on health care coverage and access?* The Commonwealth Fund. https://www.commonwealthfund.org/publications/journal-article/2020/feb/aca-at-10-years-effect-health-care-coverage-access

Brown, E. A., White, B. M., Jones, W. J., Gebregziabher, M., & Simpson, K. N. (2021, May 6). Measuring the impact of the Affordable Care Act Medicaid expansion on access to primary care using an interrupted time series approach. *Health Research Policy and Systems, 19*(77). https://health-policy-systems.biomedcentral.com/articles/10.1186/s12961-021-00730-0

Bunis, D. (2022, August 16). *Landmark bill to cut prescription drug prices signed into law.* https://www.aarp.org/politics-society/advocacy/info-2022/medicare-budget-proposal.html

Cai, A., Mehrotra, A., Germack, H. D., Busch, A. B., Huskamp, H. A., & Barnett, M. L. (2022). Trends in mental health care delivery by psychiatrists and nurse practitioners in Medicare, 2011–2019. *Health Affairs, 41*(9). https://www.healthaffairs.org/doi/abs/10.1377/hlthaff.2022.00289

Case Management Society of America (CMSA). (2021). *What is a case manager?* https://cmsa.org/who-we-are/what-is-a-case-manager/

Center for Drug Evaluation and Research. (2022, October 27). *Emergency use authorization 105* [Paxlovid]. U.S. Food and Drug Administration (FDA). https://www.fda.gov/media/155049/download

Centers for Disease Control and Prevention (CDC). (2015, March). *Invest in your community.* U.S. Department of Health and Human Services. https://www.cdc.gov/chinav/docs/chi_nav_infographic.pdf

Centers for Disease Control and Prevention (CDC). (2017, January 31). *Health disparities.* U.S. Department of Health and Human Services (HHS). https://www.cdc.gov/aging/disparities/index.htm

Centers for Disease Control and Prevention (CDC). (2020). *10 essential public health services.* U.S. Department of Health and Human Services (HHS). https://www.cdc.gov/publichealthgateway/publichealthservices/essentialhealthservices.html

Centers for Disease Control and Prevention (CDC). (2021a). *Division of Population Health at a glance.* U.S. Department of Health and Human Services. https://www.cdc.gov/chronicdisease/resources/publications/aag/population-health.htm

Centers for Disease Control and Prevention (CDC). (2022a, February 2). *What is health literacy?* U.S. Department of Health and Human Services (HHS). https://www.cdc.gov/healthliteracy/learn/index.html

Centers for Disease Control and Prevention. (CDC). (2022b, July 1). *What is health equity?* U.S. Department of Health and Human Services (HHS). https://www.cdc.gov/coronavirus/2019-ncov/community/health-equity/race-ethnicity.html

Centers for Disease Control and Prevention (CDC). (2022c, October 11). *Fast facts: Preventing intimate partner violence.* U.S. Department of Health and Human Services (HHS). https://www.cdc.gov/violenceprevention/intimatepartnerviolence/fastfact.html

Centers for Disease Control and Prevention (CDC). (2022d, October 25). *CDC community health improvement navigator.* U.S. Department of Health and Human Services. https://www.cdc.gov/chinav/index.html

Centers for Medicare and Medicaid Services (CMS). (2021, May). *Operational elements toolkit.* U.S. Department of Health and Human Services (HHS). https://innovation.cms.gov/media/document/aco-operational-elements-toolkit

Centers for Medicare and Medicaid Services (CMS). (2022a). *Accountable care organizations (ACOs): General information.* U.S. Department Health and Human Services (HHS). https://innovation.cms.gov/innovation-models/aco

Centers for Medicare and Medicaid Services (CMS). (2022b). *Home health services.* U.S. Department of Health and Human Services (HHS). https://www.medicare.gov/coverage/home-health-services

Chiara, A. (2019, March 26). *The expanding role of pharmacists: A positive shift for health care.* Commonwealth Medicine. UMass Chan Medical School. https://commed.umassmed.edu/blog/2019/03/26/expanding-role-pharmacists-positive-shift-health-care

Commonwealth Fund. (2019, April 22). *Pharmacy benefit managers and their role in drug spending*. https://www.commonwealthfund.org/publications/explainer/2019/apr/pharmacy-benefit-managers-and-their-role-drug-spending

Council on Linkages between Academia and Public Health Practice. (2021, October). *Core competencies for public health professionals*. Public Health Foundation (PHF). http://www.phf.org/resourcestools/pages/core_public_health_competencies.aspx

Creedon, T., B., Zuvekas, S. H., Hill, S. C., Ali, M. M., McClellan, C., & Dey, J. G. (2022, July 10). Effects of Medicaid expansion on insurance coverage and health services use among adults with disabilities newly eligible for Medicaid. *Health Services Research, 57*(S2), 183–194. https://onlinelibrary.wiley.com/doi/epdf/10.1111/1475-6773.14034

Day, A. M., Lewis, M. E., Meredith, R. S., Patzek, A. M., & Vogel, T. M. (2022, May). Outreach score identifies care coordination needs. *American Nurse Journal, 17*(6), 58–62. https://www.myamericannurse.com/outreach-score-identifies-care-coordination-needs/

Dolansky, M. A., & Lvisey, K. R. (2021, October). Preparing RNs for emerging roles in primary care: Shifts in care delivery require a shift in nurse preparation. *American Nurse Journal, 16*(10), 77–80.

Federal Emergency Management Agency (FEMA). (2018, June). *Engaging faith-based and community organizations: Planning considerations for emergency managers*. U.S. Department of Homeland Security (DHS). https://www.fema.gov/sites/default/files/2020-07/engaging-faith-based-and-community-organizations.pdf

Finkelman, A. (2011). *Case management for nurses*. Pearson Education.

Finkelman, A. (2021). *Professional nursing concepts: Competencies for quality leadership*. (5th ed.). Jones & Bartlett Learning.

Grant, R. (2012, June). A bridge between public health and primary care. *American Journal of Public Health, 102*(S3), S304. https://ajph.aphapublications.org/doi/full/10.2105/AJPH.2012.300825

Heath, S. (2017, September 19). *What is the difference between urgent care, retail health clinics?* Patient engagement HIT. https://patientengagementhit.com/news/what-is-the-difference-between-urgent-care-retail-health-clinics

Hirsch, L. (2022, September 5). CVS makes $8 billion bet on the r4eturn of the house call. *New York Times*. https://www.nytimes.com/2022/09/05/business/cvs-signify-health.html

HHS Press Office. (2021, October 14). *HHS announces availability of $100 million for state loan repayment programs to support primary healthcare workforce in underserved communities*. U.S. Department of Health and Human Services (HHS). https://www.hhs.gov/about/news/2021/10/14/hhs-announces-availability-100-million-state-loan-repayment-funding-to-support-health-workforce.html?utm_campaign=enews20211021&utm_medium=email&utm_source=govdelivery

HHS Press Office. (2022a, April 15). *HHS announces $226.5 million to launch community health worker training program*. U.S. Department of Health and Human Services (HHS). https://www.hhs.gov/about/news/2022/04/15/

hhs-announces-226-million-launch-community-health-worker-training-program.html

HHS Press Office. (2022b, April 21). *HHS announces $90 million to support new data-driven approaches for health centers to identify and reduce health disparities.* U.S. Department of Health and Human Services (HHS). https://www.hhs.gov/about/news/2022/04/21/hhs-announces-90-million-support-new-data-driven-approaches-health-centers-identify-reduce-health-disparities.html?utm_campaign=enews20220421&utm_medium=email&utm_source=govdelivery

HHS Press Office. (2022c, May 3). *HHS awards nearly $25 million to expand access to school-based health services.* https://www.hhs.gov/about/news/2022/05/03/hhs-awards-nearly-25-million-expand-access-school-based-health-services.html?utm_campaign=enews20220505&utm_medium=email&utm_source=govdelivery

HHS Press Office. (2022d, August 7). *News release: Statement by HHS Secretary Xavier Becerra on Senate passage of the Inflation Reduction Act.* https://www.hhs.gov/about/news/2022/08/07/statement-by-hhs-secretary-xavier-becerra-on-senate-passage-of-the-inflation-reduction-act.html

HHS Press Office. (2022e, August 8). *HHS awards nearly $90 million to community health centers to advance health equity through better data.* https://www.hhs.gov/about/news/2022/08/08/hhs-awards-nearly-90-million-dollars-to-community-health-centers-to-advance-health-equity-through-better-data.html

HHS Press Office. (2022f, August 8). *HHS invests nearly $60 million to strengthen health care workforce and improve access to care in rural communities.* https://www.hhs.gov/about/news/2022/08/08/hhs-invests-nearly-60-million-to-strengthen-health-care-workforce-and-improve-access-to-care-in-rural-communities.html?utm_campaign=enews20220818&utm_medium=email&utm_source=govdelivery

Human Resources and Services Administration (HRSA). (2021a, November). *HRSA strategic plan FY 2019–2022.* U.S. Department of Health and Human Services (HHS). https://www.hrsa.gov/about/strategic-plan/fy2019-2022

Human Resources and Services Administration (HRSA). (2021b, December). *What is a health center?* U.S. Department of Health and Human Services (HHS). https://bphc.hrsa.gov/about-health-centers/what-health-center

Human Resources and Services Administration (HRSA), (2022a, March). *Public health resources.* U.S. Department of Health and Human Services (HHS). https://www.hrsa.gov/get-health-care/resources

Human Resources and Services Administration (HRSA). (2022b, April 29). *April in Brief: HRSA works to strengthen and expand health care access.* U.S. Department of Health and Human Services (HHS). https://www.hrsa.gov/about/news/press-releases/april-2022-roundup?utm_campaign=enews20220505&utm_medium=email&utm_source=govdelivery

Human Resources and Services Administration (HRSA). (2022c, October). *Maternal, infant, and early childhood home visiting (MIECHV) program.* U.S. Department of Health and Human Services (HHS). https://mchb.hrsa.gov/programs-impact/programs/home-visiting/maternal-infant-early-childhood-home-visiting-miechv-program

International Association of Forensic Nurses (IAFN). (2022a). *Correctional nursing.* https://www.forensicnurses.org/page/CorrectionalNursing/

International Association of Forensic Nurses (IAFN). (2022b). *Sexual assault nurse examiner.* https://www.forensicnurses.org/page/aboutSANE

Institute for Healthcare Improvement (IHI). (2022a, August 18). *Prioritizing what matters most to older adults across the care continuum.* https://www.ihi.org/communities/blogs/prioritizing-what-matters-most-to-older-adults-across-the-care-continuum?utm_campaign=tw&utm_medium=email&_hsmi=223478095&_hsenc=p2ANqtz-_lSep-q7RBdczRk6KgcEqHrd23DhBNSrejtc4hVaQ5e2MCrX_blagg7BdJR8oT9mC2Aasc7BwJJKDBysfpmFraeQhiUw&utm_content=223337186&utm_source=hs_email

Institute for Healthcare Improvement (IHI). (2022b). *What is an age-friendly health system?* https://www.ihi.org/Engage/Initiatives/Age-Friendly-Health-Systems/Pages/default.aspx

International Home Care Nurses Organization (IHCNO). (2022). *International Home Care Nurses Organization.* https://ihcno.org/

John A. Hartford Foundation (JAHF) & Institute for Health Improvement (IHI). (2022, January 26). *Book: Age-friendly health systems—A guide to using the 4Ms while caring for older adults.* https://www.johnahartford.org/dissemination-center/view/book-age-friendly-health-systems-a-guide-to-using-the-4ms-while-caring-for-older-adults

Kaplan, A., Abou-sabe, K., & Nguyen, V. (2022, August 19). Frustrated pharmacists are opting out of the insurance system, saving some customers hundreds of dollars a month. *NBC News.* https://www.nbcnews.com/health/health-care/frustrated-pharmacists-are-opting-insurance-system-saving-customers-hu-rcna36706

Kates, J., Gerolamo, A., & Pogorzelska-Maziarz, M. (2021, May). The impact of COVID-19 on the hospice and palliative care workforce. *Public Health Nursing, 38*(3), 459–463. https://onlinelibrary.wiley.com/doi/10.1111/phn.12827

Landor, M., Schroeder, K., & Thompson, T-A. K. (2020). Managing care transitions to the community during a pandemic. *Journal of Nursing Administration, 50*(9), 438–441. https://journals.lww.com/jonajournal/Abstract/2020/09000/Managing_Care_Transitions_to_the_Community_During.2.aspx

Mager, N. D., & Moore, T. S. (2020, November). Healthy People 2030: roadmap for public health for the next decade. *American Journal Pharmaceutical Education, 84*(11), 8462. https://www.ajpe.org/content/84/11/8462

Malone, N. C., Williams, M. M., Fawzi, M. C. S., Bennet, J., Hill, C., Katz, J. N., & Oriol, N. E. (2020, March 20). Mobile health clinics in the United States. *International Journal of Equity Health, 19*(40). https://doi.org/10.1186/s12939-020-1135-7

Mao, A. (2022, April 28). *May is older Americans month: Elder abuse is a social determinant of health.* Office of Disease Prevention and Health Promotion.

U.S. Department of Health and Human Services (HHS). https://health.gov/news/202204/may-older-americans-month-elder-abuse-social-determinant-health?source=govdelivery&utm_medium=email&utm_source=govdelivery

Marrelli, T. (2017a, September). Caregiving and caregivers: An important part of the healthcare team. *Home Healthcare Now, 35*(8), 427–433. https://journals.lww.com/homehealthcarenurseonline/Abstract/2017/09000/Caregiving_and_Caregivers__An_Important_Part_of.5.aspx

Marrelli, T. (2017b). *A guide for caregiving: What's next?* Marrelli & Associates. https://marrelli.com/product/a-guide-for-caregiving-whats-next/

McElroy, V., Ordona, R. B., & Bakerjian, D. (2022). *Post-acute transitional services: safety in home-based care programs.* Patient Safety Network. Agency for Healthcare Research and Quality. https://psnet.ahrq.gov/primer/post-acute-transitional-services-safety-home-based-care-programs

Medicare Interactive. (2022). *Home health basics.* https://www.medicareinteractive.org/get-answers/medicare-covered-services/home-health-services/home-health-basics

Mykyta, L., Keisler-Starkey, K., & Bumch, L. (2022, September 13). *More children were covered by Medicaid and CHIP in 2021.* U.S. Census Bureau. https://www.census.gov/library/stories/2022/09/uninsured-rate-of-children-declines.html?utm_campaign=20220913msacos3ccstors&utm_medium=email&utm_source=govdelivery

National Academy of Medicine (NAM). (2018). *Making medicines affordable: A national imperative.* National Academies Press.

National Association of Community Health Centers (NACHC), Janssen Pharmaceutical Companies. (2016, August). *Population health management: Roadmap for integrated delivery networks.* http://www.nachc.org/wp-content/uploads/2015/12/NACHC_pophealth_factsheet_FINAL.pdf

National Center for Chronic Disease Prevention and Health Promotion (NCCDPHP). (2022a, July 21). *About chronic diseases.* Centers for Disease Control and Prevention. (CDC). https://www.cdc.gov/chronicdisease/about/index.htm

National Center for Chronic Disease Prevention and Health Promotion (NCCDPHP). (2022b, October 24). *Population health.* Centers for Disease Control and Prevention (CDC). https://www.cdc.gov/populationhealth/index.html

National Committee for Quality Assurance (NCQA), Janssen Pharmaceutical Companies. (2019, November). *Population health management: Roadmap for integrated delivery networks.* https://www.ncqa.org/wp-content/uploads/2019/11/20191216_PHM_Roadmap.pdf

National Institute on Aging (NIA). (2017a). *Residential facilities, assisted living, and nursing homes.* National Institutes of Health (NIH). https://www.nia.nih.gov/health/residential-facilities-assisted-living-and-nursing-homes

National Institute on Aging (NIA). (2017b). *What is long-term care?* National Institutes of Health (NIH). https://www.nia.nih.gov/health/what-long-term-care.

National Institute on Aging (NIA). (2021). *What are palliative care and hospice care?* National Institutes of Health (NIH). https://www.nia.nih.gov/health/what-are-palliative-care-and-hospice-care

National Institutes of Health (NIH). (2014, November 5). *The national prevention strategy: Prioritizing prevention to improve the nation's health.* U.S. Department of Health and Human Services (HHS). https://prevention.nih.gov/education-training/methods-mind-gap/national-prevention-strategy-prioritizing-prevention-improve-nations-health

National Institutes of Health (NIH). (2022a, July 18). *Cardiovascular-related deaths in the U.S. fall, but disparities remain.* https://www.nih.gov/news-events/news-releases/cardiovascular-related-deaths-us-fall-disparities-remain

National Institutes of Health (NIH). (2022b, August 24). *Many types of leisure time activities may lower risk of death for older adults.* U.S. Department of Health and Human Services (HHS). https://www.nih.gov/news-events/news-releases/many-types-leisure-time-activities-may-lower-risk-death-older-adults

National Institute of Nursing Research (NINR). (2022, May 6). *Introducing NINR's new strategic plan.* National Institutes of Health (NIH). https://www.ninr.nih.gov/newsandinformation/newsandnotes/strategic-plan-2022

National Institute for Occupational Safety and Health (NIOSH). (2022, June 29). *About NIOSH.* Centers for Disease Control and Prevention (CDC). https://www.cdc.gov/niosh/about/default.html

National Health Service Corps. (2022, November). *Mission, work, and impact.* Human Resources and Services Administration (HRSA). https://nhsc.hrsa.gov/about-us

Occupational Safety and Health Administration (OSHA). (2022). *OSHA.* U.S. Department of Labor (DOL). https://www.osha.gov/

Office of the Assistant Secretary for Planning and Evaluation. (2022, April 1). *HHS's strategic approach to addressing social determinants of health to advance health equity—At a glance.* U.S. Department of Health and Human Services (HHS). https://aspe.hhs.gov/sites/default/files/documents/aabf48cbd391be21e5186eeae728ccd7/SDOH-Action-Plan-At-a-Glance.pdf

Office of Disease Prevention and Health Promotion (ODPHP). (2020a). *Healthy People 2030: Browse by objectives.* U.S. Department Health and Human Services (HHS). https://health.gov/healthypeople/objectives-and-data/browse-objectives

Office of Disease Prevention and Health Promotion (ODPHP). (2020b). *Social determinants of health.* U.S. Health and Services Department (HHS). https://health.gov/healthypeople/priority-areas/social-determinants-health

Office of Disease Prevention and Health Promotion (ODPHP). (2022a, August 18). *Help us celebrate National Immunization Awareness Month!* U.S. Department Health and Human Services (HHS). https://health.gov/news/202208/help-us-celebrate-national-immunization-awareness-month

Office of Disease Prevention and Health Promotion (ODPHP). (2022b, October 6). *About ODPHP*. U.S. Department Health and Human Services (HHS). https://health.gov/about-odphp

Phillips, R. L., & Bazemore, A. W. (2010, May). Primary care and why it matters for U.S. health system reform. *Health Affairs*, *29*(5), 806–810. https://www.healthaffairs.org/doi/full/10.1377/hlthaff.2010.0020

Pitsor, J. (2022, April 18). *Bringing the benefits of telehealth to rural and underserved patients*. National Conference of State Legislatures. https://www.ncsl.org/research/health/bringing-the-benefits-of-telehealth-to-rural-and-underserved-patients-magazine2022.aspx

Quad Council Coalition Competency Review Task Force. (2018, April 13). *Community/public health nursing [C/PHN] competencies*. https://www.cphno.org/wp-content/uploads/2020/08/QCC-C-PHN-COMPETENCIES-Approved_2018.05.04_Final-002.pdf

Rural Health Information Hub (RHI Hub). (2019, June 9). *Designing age-friendly communities*. Human Resources and Services Administration (HRSA). https://www.ruralhealthinfo.org/toolkits/aging/2/age-friendly-communities

Rural Health Information Hub (RHI Hub). (2021, April 22). *Rural health clinics (RHCs)*. Human Resources and Services Administration (HRSA). https://www.ruralhealthinfo.org/topics/rural-health-clinics

Santana, S., Brach, C., Harris, L., Ochiai, E., Blakey, C., Bevington, F., Kleinman, D., & Pronk, N. (2021, November/December). Updating health literacy for Healthy People 2030: Defining its importance for a new decade in public health. *Journal of Public Health Management and Practice*, *27*(S6), S258–S264). https://journals.lww.com/jphmp/Fulltext/2021/11001/Updating_Health_Literacy_for_Healthy_People_2030_.10.aspx

Tang, M., Mehrotra, A., & Stern, A. D. (2022). Rapid growth of patient monitoring is driven by a small number of primary care providers. *Health Affairs*, *41*(9). https://www.healthaffairs.org/doi/abs/10.1377/hlthaff.2021.02026

U.S. Department of Health and Human Services (HHS). (2017, July 19). *Hospice and palliative care*. https://www.hhs.gov/guidance/document/hospice-and-palliative-care

U.S. Department of Health and Human Services (HHS). (2022, March 17). *About the Affordable Care Act*. https://www.hhs.gov/healthcare/about-the-aca/index.html

U.S. Public Health Service (USPHS). (2022). *Who we are*. U.S. Department of Health and Human Services (HHS). https://www.usphs.gov/about-us

White House. (2022, June). *Blueprint for addressing the maternal health crisis*. https://www.whitehouse.gov/wp-content/uploads/2022/06/Maternal-Health-Blueprint.pdf

World Health Organization (WHO). (2022a). *Occupational health*. https://www.who.int/health-topics/occupational-health

World Health Organization (WHO). (2022b, June 16). *World mental health report: Transforming mental health for all*. https://www.who.int/publications/i/item/9789240049338

Figure Credits

Fig. 1: Source: https://www.cdc.gov/publichealthgateway/publichealthservices/essentialhealthservices.html.

Fig. 2: Source: https://www.cdc.gov/chinav/docs/chi_nav_infographic.pdf.

Fig. 3: Source: https://www.cdc.gov/chinav/docs/chi_nav_infographic.pdf.

Fig. 4: Source: https://www.cdc.gov/chinav/docs/chi_nav_infographic.pdf.

Fig. 5: Source: https://www.cdc.gov/chinav/docs/chi_nav_infographic.pdf.

Fig. 6: Source: https://www.cdc.gov/healthyschools/parentengagement/pdf/healthy-students_badge6.pdf.

Fig. 7: Source: https://www.fema.gov/sites/default/files/2020-07/engaging-faith-based-and-community-organizations.pdf.

Fig. 8: Source: https://aspe.hhs.gov/sites/default/files/documents/aabf48cbd391be21e5186eeae728ccd7/SDOH-Action-Plan-At-a-Glance.pdf.

Fig. 9: Source: https://www.cdc.gov/chronicdisease/tools/infographics.htm.

Fig. 10: Source: https://www.ninr.nih.gov/sites/files/docs/NINR_One-Pager12_508c.pdf.

Appendix A

The National Initiative to Improve the Nation's Health: Healthy People 2030

The U.S. Department of Health and Human Services (HHS), its agencies, and other government departments are responsible for assessing and developing plans and resources to ensure the health of all people who live in the United States by promoting health and preventing disease and illness. HHS works with healthcare services at the federal, state, and local levels. Healthy People 2030 is a major federal program conducted by HHS that provides a comprehensive plan to promote health, prevent disease, and routinely assess national health status. The initiative is reviewed and updated every 10 years, with 5 past editions (1979, 1990, 2000, 2010, 2020) and the current edition, which is due to end in 2030. The latest edition's vision and major goals focus on the topics of health conditions, health behaviors, populations, settings and systems, and social determinants of health (SDOH).

Health status is determined by measuring birth and death rates, life expectancy, quality of life, morbidity from specific diseases, risk factors, use of ambulatory care and inpatient care, access to health providers and facilities and to healthcare, financing of healthcare services, health insurance coverage, and other factors. Quality of healthcare services is a complex healthcare issue that affects the health status of individuals and communities. There is not one single factor or behavior that determines outcomes, but rather multiple factors, such as genetics, lifestyle, gender, race/ethnic factors, nutrition, poverty level, education, environment, injury, violence, and unavailability or inaccessibility of quality health services.

Healthy People 2030 Framework

Vision

A society in which all people can achieve their full potential for health and well-being across the lifespan.

Mission

To promote, strengthen, and evaluate the nation's efforts to improve the health and well-being of all people.

Foundational Principles

The following foundational principles guide decisions about Healthy People 2030:

- The health and well-being of all people and communities is essential to a thriving, equitable society.
- Promoting health and well-being and preventing disease are linked efforts that encompass physical, mental, and social health dimensions.
- Investing to achieve the full potential for health and well-being for all provides valuable benefits to society.
- Achieving health and well-being requires eliminating health disparities, achieving health equity, and attaining health literacy.
- Healthy physical, social, and economic environments strengthen the potential to achieve health and well-being.
- Promoting and achieving the nation's health and well-being is a shared responsibility that is distributed across the national, state, tribal, and community levels, including the public, private, and not-for-profit sectors.
- Working to attain the full potential for health and well-being of the population is a component of decision-making and policy formulation across all sectors.

Overarching Goals

Achieving these broad and ambitious goals requires setting, working toward, and achieving a wide variety of much more specific goals. Healthy People 2030's overarching goals are to:

- Attain healthy, thriving lives and well-being, free of preventable disease, disability, injury, and premature death.
- Eliminate health disparities, achieve health equity, and attain health literacy to improve the health and well-being of all.
- Create social, physical, and economic environments that promote attaining full potential for health and well-being for all.

Office of Disease Prevention and Health Promotion (ODPHP), "Healthy People 2030 Framework," https://health.gov/healthypeople/about/healthy-people-2030-framework, 2021.

- Promote healthy development and healthy behaviors and well-being across all life stages.
- Engage leadership, key constituents, and the public across multiple sectors to take action and design policies that improve the health and well-being of all.

Plan of Action

To achieve the health and well-being of all people, relevant stakeholders need to be active partners, across the public, private, and nonprofit sectors. Healthy People conducts regular monitoring of the plan's progress. The results are made public on its website.

The Healthy People objectives are developed to meet the overall goals and are based on data and changed as needed during each 10-year cycle. This includes 8 broad outcome measures used to assess the program's vision, 355 measurable core public health objectives with 10-year targets and related evidence-based interventions, developmental goals for public health issues with interventions, and research objectives directed at public health issues for which there are no evidence-based interventions.

Healthy People 2030 focuses on individual health and on communities. It describes a healthy community as one that maintains a high quality of life and is productive and safe, provides both treatment and prevention services to all community members, maintains the necessary effective infrastructure (e.g., water, energy, roads, transportation, schools, playgrounds, and other services), and maintains a healthy environment (for example, an environment free of air and water pollution). Educational and community-based programs need to focus on preventing disease and injury, promoting and improving health, and enhancing quality of life. This view of a healthy community relates to the social determinants of health (SDOH).

To meet Healthy People goals, community programs and services must provide broad access (e.g., in schools, workplaces, healthcare facilities, and community sites) and offer prevention, monitoring, treatment, and rehabilitation services.

The Healthy People 2030 initiative not only provides a 10-year plan to improve healthcare in the United States but also monitors and reports on progress by assessing the outcome status of its goals and objectives. Data on current outcomes can be found on the Healthy People website. At the end of the 10-year period, all outcomes are evaluated and summarized. This information is then used to develop the plan for the next 10 years—the goals, objectives, and leading indicators.

Stakeholders

Many levels of government, organizations, and individuals are involved in the development, implementation, and evaluation of the Healthy People initiative. Nurses need to understand the importance stakeholders so that they can collaborate with relevant ones and advocate for healthy communities. **Figure A.1** describes the Healthy People stakeholders.

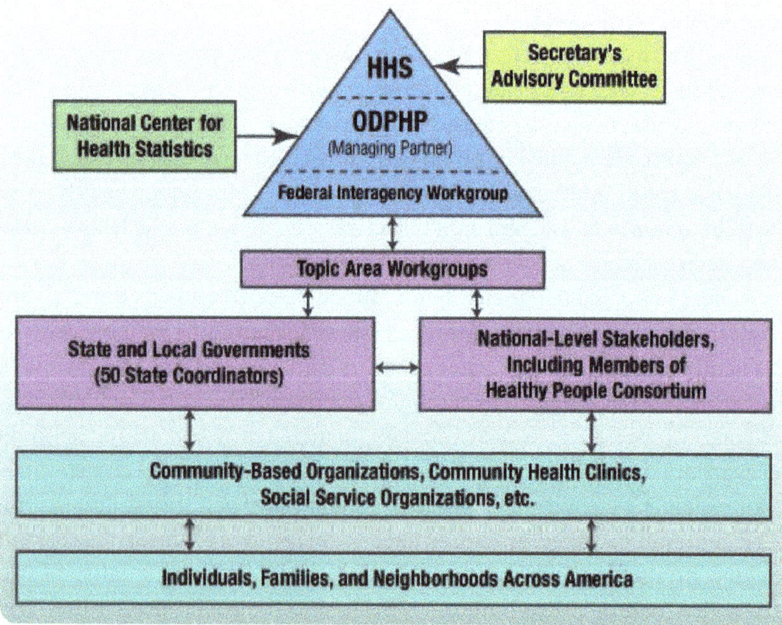

Figure A.1. Healthy People Stakeholders

Healthy People 2030: Emergency Preparedness

See information about emergency preparedness and updates on this topic at https://health.gov/healthypeople/objectives-and-data/browse-objectives/emergency-preparedness.

Healthy People 2030: Current Information

- Explore the leading health indicators used by Healthy People to monitor its outcomes.

  Source: https://health.gov/healthypeople/objectives-and-data

- Explore SDOH and their relationship to the Healthy People initiative.

  Source: https://health.gov/healthypeople/objectives-and-data

- Explore overall health and well-being measures.

  Source: https://health.gov/healthypeople/objectives-and-data

- Explore Healthy People 2030 objectives.

  Source: https://health.gov/news/202207/check-out-healthy-people-2030s-new-objectives?source=govdelivery&utm_medium=email&utm_source=govdelivery

References

Office of Disease Prevention and Health Promotion. (n.d.). *Healthy People 2030 framework*. U.S. Department of Health and Human Services (HHS). https://health.gov/healthypeople/about/healthy-people-2030-framework

Office of Disease Prevention and Health Promotion. (2021a). *Healthy People 2030*. U.S. Department of Health and Human Services (HHS). https://health.gov/healthypeople

Office of Disease Prevention and Health Promotion. (2021b). *Tools for action*. U.S. Department of Health and Human Services (HHS). https://health.gov/healthypeople/tools-action

Figure Credit

Fig. A.1: Source: https://www.cdc.gov/nchs/about/factsheets/factsheet-hp2030.htm.

Appendix B

Institute of Medicine/National Academy of Medicine Reports

The National Academy of Medicine (NAM), formerly the Institute of Medicine (IOM), examines healthcare issues and provides expert advice to healthcare organizations, individual providers, and health policymakers, both governmental and nongovernmental (NAM, 2022). The NAM is a nongovernmental, non-profit organization that was created in 1970. Why is it mentioned in this guide, which deals with equity and disparities? Its reports cover many topics, some of which are relevant to understanding health equity and disparities. The NAM asks experts to examine particular health issues, provides staff and funding for each review, and then publishes information from these reviews and often identifies recommendations (Finkelman, 2017a, 2017b). These recommendations are not laws or regulations, but they often have a major impact on healthcare policy-making.

The following are brief summaries of early reports that significantly influenced national policies of the healthcare delivery system. More current reports are also provided that highlight areas of interest covered previously.

To Err Is Human **(1999)** Due to growing questions about quality care, President William Clinton's Advisory Commission on Consumer Protection and Quality in the Health Care Industry stimulated further examination of quality and asked the IOM to further examine healthcare, focusing on errors in the healthcare delivery system. The commission's report stirred strong reaction by indicating that there were many errors in the U.S. healthcare system. The results were widely discussed in the media, so consumers became more aware of the problem. In addition, the report emphasized that the healthcare delivery system put too much emphasis on blame for errors, particularly the blame of individual staff members. This led to an active initiative to alter this approach. Most errors are system errors, not individual errors due to mistakes. The report's overall focus was acute care.

***Crossing the Quality Chasm* (2001)** A second major report on healthcare quality followed *To Err Is Human*. It focused on broader quality of care issues and concluded that more information was needed. This report also focused on acute care. Even with President Clinton's commission's review and two additional extensive reviews and reports on healthcare quality, there was still concern that we did not know enough, and the problem was more extensive. Public and community health also needed to be examined, and later reports included this vital healthcare area.

***Envisioning the National Healthcare Quality Report* (2001)** The 1999 and 2001 reports identified the need for systematic monitoring of healthcare quality to better understand the status of quality care. This monitoring needed to be done routinely and include analysis and recommendations for improvement. *Envisioning the National Healthcare Quality Report* described an initial framework for the new annual monitoring process. The Agency for Healthcare Research and Quality (AHRQ), an agency within the U.S. Department of Health and Human Services (HHS), is responsible for this annual report (titled the *National Healthcare Quality and Disparities Report*), which initially focused solely on quality care.

***Unequal Treatment: Confronting Racial and Ethnic Disparities in Health Care* (2003)** This report began to expand the healthcare perspective by analyzing disparities in public and community health. As more was learned about quality care, it became clear that there were health disparities due to bias, prejudice, and stereotyping. Just as with the issue of quality care, there was a need to monitor disparities, and this led to the development of a monitoring system and report similar to the *National Healthcare Quality and Disparities Report*, which was later combined with the quality report.

***Health Professions Education: A Bridge to Quality* (2003)** This report moved the quality care discussion to health professions education. With the growing recognition that care needed to improve and routine monitoring and was needed, it was determined that a key ingredient to accomplishing these objectives were the staff. The question was whether healthcare professionals were prepared to provide effective and efficient care to diverse populations. The report was critical in that its recommendations included five core competencies that all healthcare professionals should meet. It is significant that the experts decided to identify competencies that focused on several healthcare professions. These competencies are:

1. Provide patient-centered (or person-centered) care.
2. Work in interprofessional teams.

3. Employ evidence-based practice.
4. Apply quality improvement.
5. Utilize informatics.

Later, the nursing profession developed core competencies for nursing (Quality and Safety Education for nurses [QSEN]) that related to these core health profession competencies; however, nursing should also include the original health profession competencies. The major difference between these two types of competencies is that QSEN has six competencies and separates quality from safety, while the IOM/NAM core competencies emphasize safety as an integral part of quality.

The QSEN competencies can be reviewed at https://qsen.org/competencies/.

Health Literacy **(2004)** Aimed at examining the relationship between diversity and health disparities, the report *Health Literacy* recognized that health literacy has a major impact on quality care and the health of individuals and communities.

Health Literacy: A Prescription to End Confusion **(2004)** Communication (both written and oral) is critical in healthcare and for all stakeholders. This includes individuals, families, staff, communities, other professionals, and government agencies, among others. Effective partnerships require effective, ongoing communication. When breakdowns in communication occur, health literacy issues may arise. Understanding is necessary for effective healthcare decision-making and affections the choices of locations to obtain treatment, treatment providers, and types of treatment; the abilities to follow treatment and to engage in self-care; questions to ask healthcare providers, and so on. However, millions of Americans cannot understand or act upon this information. This report discussed health literacy and methods to improve communication for individuals and populations.

Keeping Patients Safe: Transforming the Work Environment for Nurses **(2004);** ***The Future of Nursing: Leading Change, Advancing Health*** **(2010);** ***The Future of Nursing 2020–2030: Charting a Path to Achieve Health Equity*** **(2020)** Some of the IOM/NAM reports have focused on nursing. One of the significant early reports was *Keeping Patients Safe: Transforming the Work Environment for Nurses*, which primarily discussed acute care nursing, particularly staff nurses and related workforce issues. Next a landmark report titled *The Future of Nursing: Leading Change, Advancing Health* examined current and future roles of nurses. The third report, *The Future of Nursing 2020–2030: Charting a Path to Achieve Health Equity*, is directly related to the content of this guide. All three reports are discussed in relevant sections in the guide.

***The Future of the Public's Health in the 21st Century* (2003) and *Who Will Keep the Public Healthy?* (2003)** The initial IOM reports focused on acute care, although some of the content could be applied to public and community health. There was slow recognition that separating acute care from public and community health or ignoring the healthcare delivery system as a whole was not effective. This view changed with the publication of two key public and community health reports in 2003. *The Future of the Public's Health in the 21st Century* examined the need to apply a population health approach, develop effective public health infrastructure, establish partnerships, ensure accountability, implement evidence-based practice, and utilize clear communication. *Who Will Keep the Public Healthy?* turned the focus to identifying public health competencies, which are related to informatics, genomics, communication, culture, community-based participatory research, global health, policy and law, and public health ethics. The report provided a guide for public and community health education content for many healthcare professions, such as for nursing.

***Informed Consent and Health Literacy* (2015)** This report discussed the informed consent of research participants as it related to health literacy, which by 2015 was recognized as a major concern in healthcare delivery. Research participants are asked to sign a consent form and agreeing to do so should be an informed decision. To do this, participants must understand the information they are given. Ensuring that participants can understand and give their consent prior to participating in a research study is a critical part of healthcare ethics and participant rights.

***Health Literacy: Past, Present, and Future* (2015)** Given the concern about health literacy, this report examined the problems, origins, and consequences of adult health literacy. Adults who do not have the required level of health literacy may not be able to engage safely in their own health and healthcare decision-making. The report includes proposed solutions such as the need for organizational changes, including system changes to assist in increasing health literacy.

***A Framework for Educating Health Professionals to Address Social Determinants of Health* (2016)** As more has been learned about the importance of the social determinants of health (SDOH), there has been growing recognition that healthcare professionals need to learn about these determinants so that they are more aware of their impact on health equities and disparities. Understanding the SDOH allows professional to be better able to intervene and improve the health of individuals, communities, and populations.

Collaboration Between Health Care and Public Health (2016) This report discussed the need for effective collaboration between acute health care and public health. This partnership needs to include shared goals, community engagement, aligned leadership, sustainability, and data and analysis. There are barriers to this collaboration, such inadequate communication, misunderstandings between interprofessional teams, and a lack of understanding of diverse cultures, which must be addressed in order to improve health outcomes.

Communities in Action: Pathways to Health Equity (2017) This report continued to examine health equity, disparities, and SDOH. It particularly noted that we know individual behavior and health status are important, but there is also a need to view these issues from a community perspective. It is the community that has a strong impact on poverty, unemployment, education, housing, public transportation, interpersonal violence, and struggling neighborhoods, all of which influence health. Social policies also make a difference in addressing socioeconomic and health inequality. The report examined the causes of and possible solutions to health inequities, emphasizing the importance of communities in promoting health equity.

Perspectives on Health Equity and Social Determinants of Health (2017) This report examined two social factors that influence the nation's health: racism and poverty, which result in inequitable social, environmental, and economic conditions, and health disparities. It included content on policies and strategies used to address these problems, focusing on the need for collective actions.

Community-Based Health Literacy Interventions (2018) This report focused on community interventions to reduce gaps in health literacy, examining types of community-based literacy interventions and methods to evaluate their results. It also provided examples of effective interventions. Community infrastructure and staff are critical elements to success, as is a commitment to improving community trust.

Immigration as a Social Determinant of Health (2018) The United States has a large immigrant population, which experiences systematic marginalization and discrimination that often results in health disparities. This report examined the relationship between the immigration experience and health outcomes.

Improving Access to and Equity of Care for People With Serious Illness **(2019)** At the time this report was completed, the Centers for Disease Control and Prevention (CDC) estimated that approximately 40 million people in the United States had a serious illness. An illness is considered serious if it limits daily activities. As health disparities were examined, it was noted that this population also experiences disparities due to race, ethnicity, gender, geography, socioeconomic status, and insurance status. This is found in multiple communities and interferes with healthcare access and quality. Improvement requires engagement with and feedback from individuals, families, healthcare providers, organizations, and communities.

Integrating Social Care Into the Delivery of Health Care: Moving Upstream to Improve the Nation's Health **(2019)** With the recognition of the importance of the SDOH to health equity and disparity, the healthcare delivery system must turn to improvement. The key questions addressed in this report were:

- How can services that address social needs be integrated into clinical care?
- What type of infrastructure will be needed to facilitate this integration?

The report concluded that five complementary activities should be used to ensure integration of social care into health care: awareness, adjustment, assistance, alignment, and advocacy. The report discussed these activities and stated that they should be used by healthcare organizations and providers, communities, social services, and governments.

Population Health in Rural America **(2020)** Rural areas of the United States experience many health problems and difficulty receiving effective and timely health care. People who live in rural areas are a vulnerable and diverse population. Rural areas also experience serious healthcare delivery problems, such as a shortage of healthcare professionals and services.

Population Health in Challenging Times: Insights From Key Domains, Proceedings of a Workshop **(2021)** This report examined population health, which is a complex area of health care. The workshop identified key areas of concern in population health, supporting the recognition that population health is critical to overall national health.

Priorities on the Health Horizon: Informing PCORI's Strategic Plan **(2021)** This report discussed the need for more evidence to support healthcare delivery and practice. It particularly focused on equitable, stakeholder-driven, evidence-guided, patient-centered care. All of this requires effective collaborative relationships between patients, families, clinicians, healthcare administrators, researchers, and policymakers. PCORI is the Patient-Centered Outcomes Research Institute, an independent non-profit organization in Washington, DC, authorized by Congress since 2010 to address the gaps in information needed to make effective healthcare decisions. For more information, visit https://www.pcori.org/about/about-pcori.

Dialogue About the Workforce for Population Health Improvement: Proceedings of a Workshop (2021) This workshop focused on the needs of the population health workforce to improve health. Some of the workforce groups discussed were peer-to-peer chronic disease management educators, health navigators, community health workers, and public health and healthcare leaders. The report also focused on developing competencies of the nonmedical and nonpublic health workforce and applying the health in all policies model.

Exploring the Role of Critical Health Literacy in Addressing the Social Determinants of Health: Proceedings of a Workshop in Brief (2021) Due to the growing concern about the SDOH, a discussion and subsequent report focused on this issue. It particularly addressed the impact of health literacy on SDOH and vulnerable populations. The emphasis was on using health literacy strategies to support a greater understanding of the SDOH.

To Achieve Health Equity, Leverage Nurses and Increase Funding for School and Public Health Nursing (2022) This report focused on nursing, but rather than discussing acute care, it examined the roles of nursing in public health, driven by the need to improve health equity. The key recommendations for the next 10 years included the following:

- strengthening nursing education
- promoting diversity, inclusivity, and equity in nursing education and the workforce
- investing in school and public health nurses
- protecting nurses' health and well-being
- preparing nurses for disaster and public health emergency response
- increasing the number of PhD-prepared nurses

Reducing Inequalities Between Lesbian, Gay, Bisexual, Transgender, and Queer Adolescents and Cisgender, Heterosexual Adolescents: Proceedings of a Workshop (2022) LGBTQ+ adolescents are at risk for health and social problems, and face health inequity compared to the cisgender, heterosexual peers. As a vulnerable population, they require assessment and interventions that address health equity and reduce disparities. This report examined these concerns.

Realizing the Promise of Equity in the Organ Transplantation System (2022) Organ transplantation is a complex health need supported by a complex system. A key concern is health equities and disparities for some who need this care. This report discussed the many issues patients and families experience and the system that supports organ transplantation.

Closing Evidence Gaps in Clinical Prevention (2022) This report discussed the need for more research to determine evidence-based practices in clinical prevention. The report was a collaboration between the U.S. Department of Health and Human Services and U.S. Preventive Services Task Force. For more information, visit https://www.ahrq.gov/cpi/about/otherwebsites/uspstf/index.html.

Measuring Sex, Gender Identity, and Sexual Orientation (2022) This report explored current information on the topics of sex, gender identity, and sexual orientation. An understanding of these factors is important to gaining insights into health inequities based on them.

Healthy, Resilient, and Sustainable Communities After Disasters (2015) Communities must recover after disasters and work with multiple stakeholders to rebuild and repair infrastructure, provide health and social services, and provide new resources. Equitable access is a critical element.

Community Power in Population Health Improvement (2022) Community power is required to assess and improve population health within a community. This report discussed various actions that might be taken. Examples of topics included were education, transportation, environmental health, healthy eating, and active living.

Rapid Expert Consultation on Crisis Standards of Care for the COVID-19 Pandemic (2021) Crisis standards of care are not new, but during the COVID-19 pandemic more consumers and healthcare providers and organizations became familiar with them and their implications. They were applied in many states and had an impact on who received care and when. Issues related to these standards of care were examined in the report.

Lessons Learned in Health Professions Education During the COVID-19 Pandemic, Parts 1 and 2 (2021; 2022) This report examined the issues and challenges that healthcare professions education confronted during the COVID-19 pandemic. Experts discussed the experience and made recommendations that should apply across a variety of healthcare professions.

Implementing High-Quality Primary Care: Rebuilding the Foundation of Health Care (2021) High-quality primary care is important for an effective healthcare system. It should provide continuous, person-centered, relationship-based care that considers the needs and preferences of individuals, families, and communities. Primary care is necessary to prevent health problems from becoming more serious, reducing the need for more extensive healthcare services and reducing costs.

Integrating the Patient and Caregiver Voice in Serious Illness (2017) This report discussed the need for overall care quality through the delivery of person-centered and family-oriented services, for patients of all ages and across disease stages, care settings, and specialties. The increasing number of older adults represent a vulnerable population that requires health system support and other services to meet their complex needs. However, other complex needs can be found across the age spectrum and in a broad range of care settings, from perinatal care to geriatric care.

Caring for People With Serious Illness: Lessons Learned From the COVID-19 Pandemic (2022) This report discussed the impact of the COVID-19 pandemic, noting ongoing weaknesses in the U.S. healthcare system and the need to address challenges related to caring for people with serious illness. Some of the issues included in this discussion included the legal liability of healthcare teams providing care to people with serious illness, the impact of the pandemic on the healthcare workforce, the use of telehealth, issues related to clearly communicating with the public about health emergencies, policy opportunities to improve care for people with serious illness, and health equity.

Models for Population Health Improvement by Health Care Systems and Partners: Tensions and Promise on the Path Upstream (2022) The CDC reevaluated many of its current disease control mechanisms, including the use and role of quarantine as a public health tool. This report was part of this reevaluation. The report recommended that assessments of disease control efficacy should consider disease management responsibilities and the federal quarantine station network in mitigating the risk of onward communicable disease transmission while considering changes in the global environment, including large increases in international travel, threats posed by emerging infections, and the movement of animals and cargo.

Examples of Other Reports

- *Collaboration Between Health Care and Public Health* (2015)
- *The Future of Home Health Care* (2015)
- *Health Literacy: Past, Present, and Future* (2015)
- *Informed Consent and Health Literacy* (2015)
- *Community-Based Health Literacy Interventions* (2018)
- *Improving Access to and Equity of Care for People With Serious Illness* (2019)
- *Integrating Social Care into the Delivery of Health Care: Moving Upstream to Improve the Nation's Health* (2019)
- *A Roadmap to Reducing Childhood Poverty* (2019)
- *School Success: An Opportunity for Population Health* (2019)
- *Virtual Clinical Trials: Challenges and Opportunities* (2019)
- *Faith Health Collaboration to Improve Community and Population Health* (2021)
- *The National Imperative to Improve Nursing Home Quality: Honoring Our Commitment to Residents, Families, and Staff* (2021)
- *Population Health in Rural America in 2020* (2021)
- *Emerging Stronger From COVID-19: Priorities for Health System Transformation* (2022)
- *Evolving Crisis Standards of Care and Ongoing Lessons From COVID-19* (2022)
- *Improving the CDC Quarantine Station Network's Response to Emerging Threats* (2022)

Access to IOM/NAM Reports

NAM publishes many reports annually. The reports and other IOM/NAM resources can be read online or downloaded for free using the guest status. Full or partial reports can be reviewed. There is no fee to access these reports. This information can be accessed at https://nam.edu/publications/.

References

Finkelman, A. (2017a). *Teaching the IOM: Implications of the IOM Reports for Nursing Education* (1st vol., 4th ed.). American Nurses Association.

Finkelman, A. (2017b). *Learning IOM: Adapted content for students and staff* (2nd vol., 4th ed.). American Nurses Association.

National Academcy of Medicine. (2022). About. Retrieved from https://nam.edu/about-the-nam/

Quality and Safety Education for Nurses (QSEN) Institute. (2020). *QSEN Institute competencies*. https://qsen.org/competencies/

Index

K

L

M

N

O

P

About the Author

Anita Finkelman, MSN, RN is a nurse educator and consultant, currently providing services in the U.S. and Israel, where she has been visiting faculty at Recanati School for Community Health Professions at Ben-Gurion University of the Negev and consulted with several Israeli universities. She served on the nursing faculty at Bouvé College of Health Sciences, School of Nursing, Northeastern University, where she taught undergraduate and graduate online courses and led the nursing school's CCNE accreditation process for undergraduate and graduate programs with full accreditation received. She previously served as an assistant professor of nursing at the University of Oklahoma College of Nursing, where she taught undergraduate and graduate nursing online courses and served as course coordinator for undergraduate nursing research. At the University of Cincinnati, Finkelman was an associate professor of clinical nursing, the director of continuing education, and the director of the undergraduate program (BSN), and taught public/community health, mental health nursing, nursing leadership, health policy, research courses, and clinical practicum. She has worked with several smaller colleges to develop and implement online programs and develop curriculum for pre-licensure nursing students.

Finkelman earned her BSN from Texas Christian University and her master's degree in psychiatric-mental health nursing/clinical nurse specialist from Yale University. She completed post-master's graduate work in healthcare policy and administration at George Washington University and participated as a fellow in the Health Policy Institute at George Mason University. Her nursing experience includes clinical, educational, and administrative positions and considerable experience developing distance education programs and curriculum, as well as a long history of teaching online. Finkelman has extensive management experience serving in various positions in psychiatric-mental health settings (acute care and community), having served as the director of staff education for two acute care hospitals and within clinical nurse specialist positions. As a consultant, she focuses on areas of curriculum and quality improvement, teaching-learning practices, distance education, healthcare administration and policy, nursing education accreditation, and assisting nurses in their publishing endeavors.

She has authored many books, chapters, and journal articles, served on journal editorial boards, and made presentations on nursing education, healthcare administration, health policy, healthcare quality improvement, continuing education, and psychiatric-mental health nursing, both nationally and internationally. She serves as a consultant to publishers in the areas of distance education and product development.

Finkelman's textbooks include *Professional Nursing Concepts* (Jones and Bartlett Learning, 5th ed., 2021); *Quality Improvement: A Guide for Integration in Nursing*, (Jones & Bartlett Learning, 2nd ed., 2020); *Leadership and Management for Nurses: Core Competencies for Quality Care* (Pearson Education, Inc., 4th ed., 2020); and *Case Management for Nurses* (Pearson Education, Inc., 2010). She has also authored chapters in M. Nies and M. McEwen's (Eds.) *Community Health Nursing: Promoting the Health of Aggregates*, Philadelphia, PA: W. B. Saunders Company.

www.ingramcontent.com/pod-product-compliance
Ingram Content Group UK Ltd.
Pitfield, Milton Keynes, MK11 3LW, UK
UKHW021830270726
14058UKWH00001B/61